The Multiple Sclerosis Diet Book

Tessa Buckley worked as an architectural assistant and interior designer in London, until a diagnosis of multiple sclerosis cut short her career. She is now a freelance writer, specializing in the fields of health and nutrition and family history. She also writes novels for children. She has two grown-up children and lives by the sea in Essex with her husband, a retired teacher. You can find out more about Tessa and her books at <www.tessabuckley.com>.

D1419682

4 1 0275885 3

Overcoming Common Problems Series

Selected titles

A full list of titles is available from Sheldon Press,
36 Causton Street, London SW1P 4ST and on our website at
www.sheldonpress.co.uk

Beating Insomnia: Without really trying
Dr Tim Cantopher

Birth Over 35
Sheila Kitzinger

Breast Cancer: Your treatment choices
Dr Terry Priestman

Chronic Fatigue Syndrome: What you need to know about CFS/ME
Dr Megan A. Arroll

The Chronic Pain Diet Book
Neville Shone

Cider Vinegar
Margaret Hills

Coeliac Disease: What you need to know
Alex Gazzola

Coping Successfully with Chronic Illness: Your healing plan
Neville Shone

Coping Successfully with Hiatus Hernia
Dr Tom Smith

Coping Successfully with Pain
Neville Shone

Coping Successfully with Panic Attacks
Shirley Trickett

Coping Successfully with Prostate Cancer
Dr Tom Smith

Coping Successfully with Shyness
Margaret Oakes, Professor Robert Bor and Dr Carina Eriksen

Coping Successfully with Ulcerative Colitis
Peter Cartwright

Coping Successfully with Varicose Veins
Christine Craggs-Hinton

Coping Successfully with Your Irritable Bowel
Rosemary Nicol

Coping with a Mental Health Crisis: Seven steps to healing
Catherine G. Lucas

Coping with Anaemia
Dr Tom Smith

Coping with Asthma in Adults
Mark Greener

Coping with Blushing
Professor Robert J. Edelmann

Coping with Bronchitis and Emphysema
Dr Tom Smith

Coping with Chemotherapy
Dr Terry Priestman

Coping with Coeliac Disease: Strategies to change your diet and life
Karen Brody

Coping with Difficult Families
Dr Jane McGregor and Tim McGregor

Coping with Diverticulitis
Peter Cartwright

Coping with Dyspraxia
Jill Eckersley

Coping with Early-onset Dementia
Jill Eckersley

Coping with Endometriosis
Jill Eckersley and Dr Zara Aziz

Coping with Envy: Feeling at a disadvantage with friends and family
Dr Windy Dryden

Coping with Epilepsy
Dr Pamela Crawford and Fiona Marshall

Coping with Gout
Christine Craggs-Hinton

Coping with Guilt
Dr Windy Dryden

Coping with Headaches and Migraine
Alison Frith

Coping with Heartburn and Reflux
Dr Tom Smith

Coping with Life after Stroke
Dr Mareeni Raymond

Coping with Liver Disease
Mark Greener

Coping with Memory Problems
Dr Sallie Baxendale

Coping with Obsessive Compulsive Disorder
Professor Kevin Gournay, Rachel Piper and Professor Paul Rogers

Coping with Pet Loss
Robin Grey

Coping with Phobias and Panic
Professor Kevin Gournay

Overcoming Common Problems

The Multiple Sclerosis Diet Book

TESSA BUCKLEY

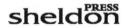

First published in Great Britain in 2017

Sheldon Press
36 Causton Street
London SW1P 4ST
www.sheldonpress.co.uk

British Library Cataloguing-in-Publication Data
A catalogue record for this book is available from the British Library

ISBN 978–1–84709–415–5
eBook ISBN 978–1–84709–416–2

Typeset by Fakenham Prepress Solutions, Fakenham, Norfolk NR21 8NN
First printed in Great Britain by Ashford Colour Press
Subsequently digitally printed in Great Britain

eBook by Fakenham Prepress Solutions, Fakenham, Norfolk NR21 8NN

Produced on paper from sustainable forests

In memory of my mother, who was the first person to demonstrate to me that some foods can make you ill and some foods can make you better.

Contents

Acknowledgements

I am grateful to Mark Greener for helping to elucidate some knotty scientific jargon, and to *New Pathways* magazine, published by MS-UK, as its informative articles on nutritional therapy and MS pointed the way for much of my own research. Thanks also to all the people who took the time to tell me about their experiences with MS diets, especially the six who allowed their stories to be used as case studies.

Note to the reader

This is not a medical book and is not intended to replace advice from your doctor. Consult your pharmacist or doctor if you believe you have any of the symptoms described, and if you think you might need medical help.

Preface to the new edition

Since I finished writing *The Multiple Sclerosis Diet Book* in 2006, research into the causes and treatment of multiple sclerosis (MS) has produced a great deal of new and useful information. However, at the time of writing there are still no tried, tested and clinically proven drug treatments available for those with progressive MS, and treatments for relapsing–remitting MS do not claim to do more than slow down the rate of relapses. Therefore nutritional therapy remains, as it has been in the past, a useful self-help option to try.

Two new diets for MS have emerged over the last few years: the Overcoming MS diet, and the Wahls diet, and I cover both of these in this new edition. We also know a lot more than we did a few years ago about the importance of vitamin D and omega-3 fatty acids to the health of both the general public and those with MS. New information on both the benefits and the dangers of some vitamins and minerals has emerged, and research confirming the adverse effects of substances such as salt and sugar for people with MS has been published. At the same time, the anecdotal evidence from people with MS (including health professionals) who have benefited from changing their eating habits has continued to appear.

As you will see from some of the case studies, changing your diet can be helpful even if you are also taking disease-modifying drugs, and many people go on to make additional life changes such as practising meditation or taking regular exercise. Professor George Jelinek goes even further. He suggests in his book *Overcoming Multiple Sclerosis* that for some people, making lifestyle modifications such as changing your diet may be more useful than taking drugs when dealing with chronic diseases such as MS.

In the 26 years since I was diagnosed with progressive MS, I have never taken (or been offered) any disease-modifying drugs and yet, at an age when most of my friends are retiring and starting to slow down, I am more energetic than ever, writing and getting involved with community activities. I put my present energy and relative stability down to following a strict diet, taking a few key supplements and exercising regularly to prevent muscle deterioration.

I hope that reading this book will show you how important food is to our health, and maybe encourage you to experiment with one of the diets to see if it will benefit you. The recipes are designed to be tasty and simple to make as well as nutritionally balanced, because meals should be enjoyable even if you are on a special diet. *Bon appétit* – and good health!

Introduction: my story

When I was young, the two things that caused me the most health problems were stress and food. As a child, even 'good' stress, such as the excitement of going on holiday, always gave me tummy upsets. Stress has also always made me vulnerable to viruses and infections, and a particularly stressful event that occurred when I was 12 precipitated a bout of glandular fever. Some foods also made me ill. For instance, by the age of 10 I had already worked out that the reason I felt so ill each Easter was that chocolate eggs disagreed with me. I hated the taste of milk, too, and drinking my daily quota at school each day often made me feel sick. Sweet, sugary foods also made me feel queasy.

Throughout my childhood I watched my mother struggling with irritable bowel syndrome, which was very poorly understood in the 1960s. She did a lot of research into nutrition and eventually worked out that if she avoided fried food, pork, tomatoes, oranges and onions, she could keep her symptoms under control. Her doctor couldn't explain why avoiding certain foods worked, though, and it wasn't until we came across Dr Richard Mackarness' book *Not All in the Mind* (Pan, 1976) in the 1970s that we discovered that food intolerance offered a possible explanation for our problems with food. But although I'd given up chocolate and rarely ate sweets, I continued to eat dairy products – I wasn't ready to give them up yet.

In 1971 I left home and went to college to study interior design. Good student accommodation was difficult to find in London, and I ended up living in a house run by a racketeering landlord and full of petty criminals. Although I eventually found a safer place to live and moved out, the stress of it all proved too much for me, and I began to suffer from lack of confidence and panic attacks. After I'd completed my final exams I also experienced a brief period of blurred vision, which my doctor attributed – unsurprisingly – to stress. She suggested I should do something that would help me relax, so I started practising yoga and meditation.

When I left college, interior design jobs were in short supply but I managed to find work as an architectural assistant. Through a combination of luck and hard work, by the time I was 30 I was running a multimillion-pound building project in central London. I had got married, too, and was supporting my husband, Gwyn, through university while he trained as a teacher. The stresses in both my work and my marriage were building, and 1980 was a crunch year for us. We both needed to relax and spend some quality time together, so we set off on a trip to Paris and the Loire Valley. It was a wonderful holiday, but on the way home I started to feel ill. My muscles and glands all ached and I had a virulent sore throat. 'Some sort of virus,' said my GP. 'Take a week off work and rest.'

From then on, I got similar viruses at least once a year. By 1984, I was feeling stressed out again and I had constant tension in my neck and shoulders. I was so tired that it was difficult to function at work, let alone have a social life. I wondered if exercise would perk me up, and decided to try aerobics. It was a disaster. After 20 minutes of non-stop exercise, I ended up curled up on the floor like a dead fly with all my muscles in spasm and a circle of concerned faces looking down on me. 'Panic attack,' said my GP when I told him about it. 'Lack of CO_2. Next time it happens, try breathing into a paper bag.' The attacks continued, and I began to fear what would happen if I had one when I was on a building site – not the safest of places at the best of times. I discussed the situation with Gwyn and we decided we had enough savings to support us for three months, so I handed in my notice and started to review my life.

I re-read *Not All in the Mind* and started to see a pattern emerging. I don't normally drink coffee, but when I was doing my finals at college I had taken tablets called Pro Plus, which contained concentrated caffeine, so I could stay awake and get more work done. When we were in France I had been seduced by the smell of freshly percolated black coffee and had drunk gallons of it. Could the Pro Plus have sensitized me to caffeine so that now I could no longer tolerate it? Perhaps if I avoided caffeine from now on I wouldn't get any more viruses. I decided to cut out coffee and tea and see what happened. Then I remembered all my problems with chocolate, how I'd hated milk, and how cream cakes always disagreed with me. It was definitely time to give up dairy products.

That was a turning point for me. My energy returned and I no longer had permanently aching shoulders. After a long rest and feeling better than I had in ages, I returned to work.

Six months later, out of the blue, I was made redundant. My stress levels started rising again as I struggled to keep us afloat financially, moving from job to job for the next couple of years. At the same time, things started to go wrong in my life. I fell out with my best friend; I was told I'd probably never have children; and my father died. Then, while we were on holiday in Spain, I had an episode where I felt as if I was having a heart attack. However, after I'd rested for a bit I felt much better, so I managed to put the whole thing out of my mind.

In February 1987, to my amazement and delight, I found I was pregnant, and in August of that year I gave birth to my first child, Louise. Although the birth itself was relatively easy, from then on I never really felt 100 per cent. It didn't occur to me that anything major could be wrong; I thought it was just exhaustion caused by interrupted nights and adjusting to becoming a mother. I was making plans to return to work when I started to have problems with my bowels. Embarrassingly, they would open without warning so that sometimes I wouldn't make it to the toilet in time. So it was back to our GP, who referred me to the coeliac unit at our local hospital where, after various tests, I was diagnosed with coeliac disease and put on a gluten-free diet for life.

I had barely got used to the new diet when my legs started to play up. I had a pain like sciatica in my hip and my leg dragged when I walked. Sometimes my ankles would give out and I couldn't walk far before I needed a rest. I was referred to a neurologist, still blissfully unaware that anything serious was wrong, so it came as quite a shock when he told me he was about 95 per cent certain that I had multiple sclerosis. This was 1988 and disease-modifying drugs were still a long way in the future. 'There's nothing we can do for you at present,' he said. 'Read as much about MS as you can, then at least you'll be prepared for what's to come.'

The only book I could find on MS was *MS: A self-help guide to its management* by Judy Graham (Healing Arts Press, 1981). The consultant had said that diet wouldn't help, yet Judy Graham was advocating a low-fat diet. I remembered how my mother had proved you could treat yourself with diet despite being pooh-poohed by her doctors, so I decided to give it a try.

By now my diet was dairy-free, gluten-free, caffeine-free and low-fat. I also consulted a doctor of nutritional medicine. He recommended I take vitamins A, C, E and B complex, zinc and selenium. He then used kinesiology to test me for food intolerances and suggested that I omit orange juice, nuts and eggs from my diet for a couple of months, before reintroducing them on an occasional basis.

Nothing much changed until, about six months later, I woke up one morning and noticed that I felt different. Normally dragging myself out of bed in the morning was a huge chore but now I couldn't wait to get up. I even did some yoga before breakfast. Gwyn and I met friends for lunch, and the walk from the station to the restaurant suddenly wasn't a problem. Could this be a remission? I continued to feel so much better that I persuaded a local architect to employ me four days a week and was soon back at work. In retrospect, I probably tried to do too much too soon. The work was easy, but it was a hot summer and I had a young child to look after. After six happy weeks, I started to go downhill again.

Then two things happened at once. I found I was pregnant again, and Gwyn was offered the chance to change places with a teacher in Australia for a year. He'd grown up in Adelaide and wanted to go back and see old friends. It was a tough decision, but I felt if I didn't go then, I might not be able to go in the future. In the event it was a wonderful experience. We lived in a small town on the north coast of Tasmania in a large house overlooking the sea, and our son Patrick was born there in May 1990. I had help from social services and the local MS society, and we managed to visit friends and family on the mainland. In January 1991 when we flew back from an Australian summer to a British winter, it was quite a shock to the system.

By this stage it was obvious that I wasn't going to be able to return to work and that I would need help looking after the children until they were old enough to go to school. I continued on the diet and supplements, but although I had plenty of energy and wasn't developing any fresh symptoms, my walking was still deteriorating. I felt diet alone wasn't going to be enough to halt the decline, so I followed up a tip I'd been given in Australia about a clinic in London that advocated weightlifting for people with MS. Using large machines called leg presses, the trainees lay on their backs and lifted the weights with their feet. The theory was that putting pressure on the spine like this had a positive effect on the nervous system. In fact it was a very convenient way of exercising for anyone who couldn't run or do continuous repetitive movements. I'm quite small and slight, and I could never lift as much as the other trainees, but I persevered and after two years my condition seemed to stabilize. I carried on exercising for another 18 months until we left London and moved to Essex in 1994. Since then, diet has been the only form of therapy I've used, although I have continued to exercise regularly using exercises devised for me by a physiotherapist and personal trainer.

In 2003 I heard for the first time how the symptoms of Hughes Syndrome could mimic MS, and I asked my GP if I could be tested for Hughes, as no doctor had ever been 100 per cent sure that I had MS. The blood test came back positive, and my consultant suggested I should spend five days in hospital having tests to obtain a definitive diagnosis. Since Hughes Syndrome is treatable with warfarin, I was hoping to swap my diagnosis of MS for one of Hughes. I should have known it wouldn't be that simple. The lumbar puncture and MRI scan confirmed I had MS, but the blood tests showed unmistakeably that I had Hughes Syndrome too. I had just gained a third chronic medical condition.

For 13 years, from 1994 until 2007, my MS symptoms remained stable. Then in 2007 I had a fall and broke my leg, and this led to some disease progression and the discovery that I had osteoporosis. I now use a wheelchair when outside the home as I don't want to risk another damaging fall, but a regular exercise routine has kept me on my feet indoors.

My diet has evolved over the years, and now my breakfasts and lunches are largely vegan, although I still eat fish, chicken and a small amount of red meat at dinner. A lot of the food we eat is organic, including much of our fruit and vegetables, which we grow on our allotment, and we buy our meat and poultry from a local butcher who sells grass-fed meat and free-range chickens. I'm still avoiding gluten, dairy products, caffeine, chocolate and sugar, and I recently had to give up eating onions, leeks and soya, but I do have the occasional glass of wine on special occasions. I also now put more emphasis on adding as many nutrient-rich foods to my diet as possible.

It is hard sometimes sticking to the diet, but I believe the results are worth it, and I enjoy cooking. Although I still do miss cheese sandwiches and cups of tea, most of the time I really enjoy the food I eat. It makes me feel good mentally, emotionally and physically, and you can't ask for more than that.

I hope that this book will help others with MS to achieve a better quality of life. As you can see from my experience, adapting your diet can make you feel better, although the exact results will vary from person to person. Why not give it a try? It may take a little time to adjust your shopping and food preparation habits, but remember – perseverance and experimentation pay off where diet is concerned. Good luck!

Part 1
FOOD AS MEDICINE

1

Food and MS

What is MS?

Multiple sclerosis is a disease that affects the central nervous system. The nerve fibres in the brain and spinal cord are surrounded by an insulating layer called the myelin sheath. What happens in MS is that the myelin breaks down, disrupting the electrical signals being transmitted along the nerves to other parts of the body, and scars or 'plaques' develop on the damaged nerves. These are the white areas that show up on MRI scans.

MS is thought to be an autoimmune disease. This means that, instead of defending the body against attack from foreign bodies such as bacteria, the immune system starts to attack healthy tissue.

However, current research suggests that there is no single cause of MS, and that it develops because of a combination of genetic and environmental factors. Some environmental factors that are actively being investigated at present as possible triggers are vitamin D deficiency, smoking and viruses.

The illness tends to affect everyone differently and causes a vast array of symptoms, only some of which will be present in each person. It is this unpredictability that frustrates doctors and patients alike. Most doctors agree, however, that there are three distinct types of MS.

- **Relapsing–remitting** In this type, there are periodic attacks, when symptoms are exacerbated, interspersed with remissions, when the symptoms disappear or die down, although each attack may leave the person marginally more disabled.
- **Primary progressive** In this case, the disease is progressive from the start, with no periods of remission, although the progress may be slow.
- **Secondary progressive** The person starts off having relapsing–remitting MS and then, after a period of time, the illness becomes progressive.

Although important gaps in our knowledge still exist concerning the cause of MS, it has been possible to develop some drugs, such as Betaferon and Copaxone, that can affect the course of the illness for people with relapsing–remitting MS. At the time of writing, however, there are still very few treatments available that will modify the course of the illness for people with primary or secondary progressive MS, although several new therapies are currently in the process of development.

How can changing your diet help MS?

This book explains how to use diet to help fight MS, an approach known as nutritional therapy.

Doctors who practise orthodox medicine use drugs, not food, to treat illness. Often, the more serious the illness, the stronger the drugs. But for some conditions – particularly degenerative diseases such as MS – even the most advanced modern drugs cannot provide a cure. The best that can be hoped for is to manage the illness using disease-modifying drugs. Drugs may also have the drawback of producing adverse side effects.

Nutritional therapists (that is, doctors of environmental, allergic and nutritional medicine, clinical ecologists, nutritionists and naturopaths), however, take a different approach to healing. They believe that what we eat and drink has a profound effect on our well-being and see symptoms of an illness as a warning that our body's biochemistry is disturbed due to three possible causes:

1 a shortage of nutrients (substances such as vitamins, minerals and essential fatty acids, or, EFAs);
2 the body's inability to absorb these nutrients properly;
3 internal pollution from chemicals either in food or the environment.

Eating foods containing the right nutrients in the right amounts can help alleviate the symptoms of disease, protect against other illnesses, and assist in healing the body and mind. Sometimes additional vitamin and mineral supplements also form part of the treatment.

To put it simply, food acts as fuel, enabling our metabolism to function properly. Our body is like the engine of a car: we have to give it the right type of fuel if we want it to perform well.

The unpredictability of MS makes people feel powerless, but there is evidence that people who feel involved in the management of their illness are more optimistic about the future than those who are not, which in turn has a positive effect on their health. Changing your diet is something you can do for yourself to help manage your symptoms. The dietary approach is not a 'cure' for MS but, as many people who have used food as medicine can testify, it can help dampen down your symptoms, raise energy levels, lift your mood, improve your general health and generate a feeling of well-being. It may also help slow down the progress of the disease, letting you stay mobile for longer.

Nutritional therapy

Nutritional therapy is a relatively new science, but a huge amount of research has already been carried out in the field, and scientists now understand a great deal about how the body uses nutrients. They have isolated 50 essential factors that the body needs to grow, to stay healthy and to repair damage, including vitamins, minerals, amino acids, essential fatty acids, starches, water, oxygen and light. These essential nutrients are team players. A shortage of any one could damage your health. The foods that contain these essential factors are the foods that heal us. Other foods, such as saturated fats, are harmful to us if we eat too much of them.

The evidence that diet affects MS

The number of trials so far on diet and MS is quite small, and not all of them have been randomized double-blind trials, the only sort that most doctors regard as scientifically valid. Trials also need to be repeated several times before the case is considered to be scientifically proven, as a positive result from a single trial could be the result of chance. Nevertheless, some of the tests done on fats and MS, while not conclusive, do strongly suggest that a diet low in saturated fat but high in certain types of EFAs might be useful. These trials are detailed on pages 46–8.

As well as research involving people with MS, there is also epidemiological evidence (statistics showing where in the world MS is most common). As these statistics can be interpreted in different ways, the following facts are not proof that diet is a factor in MS, but they strongly suggest that it might be.

- MS is a disease of temperate zones (northern Europe and North America, for example) and is virtually non-existent in the tropics.
- MS is most prevalent in places where there is a lot of dairy farming and wheat production, and least prevalent where the diet is based on fish and vegetable oils.
- In countries such as Norway, which has a long coastline, more people with MS live in inland areas, where the diet is high in dairy products, and fewer in coastal areas, where a lot of fish is eaten.
- MS increases in frequency the further you travel from the equator. This suggests there may be a link with lack of vitamin D, as the main source of this vitamin is sunlight. The other source of vitamin D is fish, which is eaten in large quantities in areas where there is a low occurrence of MS.
- Israel and the West Indies both have a relatively low incidence of MS. However, people who emigrated to Israel from northern Europe are more likely to have MS than those who were born in Israel. Similarly, people who emigrated to the UK from the West Indies have a much higher rate of MS than those who stayed there. This suggests that they may have been affected by a change in diet.

In addition to clinical trials and epidemiological studies, there is plenty of anecdotal evidence from people who have used various diets as aids to recovery. Two of the pioneers in this field were Roger MacDougall and Alan Greer, both of whom used exclusion diets to halt or reverse the progress of their MS.

The playwright Roger MacDougall devised his own diet for MS after being diagnosed in 1953. He eventually found that by reducing saturated fats, excluding gluten, sugar and most dairy products, and supplementing with polyunsaturated fatty acids (PUFAs) and vitamins and minerals, he could halt and even reverse his decline. He lived into his eighties and was still mobile at the time of his death.

Alan Greer was another person who benefited hugely from changing his diet. His wife, Rita, first realized that Alan seemed to be sensitive to certain common foods and began to experiment with his diet. Alan seemed to have strong allergic reactions to foods, so it was quite easy to identify the culprits. The list of foods Alan eventually gave up included meat, dairy products, gluten and eggs, and for the first four years he ate an essentially vegan diet. He also exercised daily. After a while his condition had improved so much that people began to question his original diagnosis. Then in 1992 he had major surgery to remove a brain tumour, and had to spend a long time in hospital and subsequently in a nursing home, recovering. He no longer had access to a specialized diet, and after a year all his MS symptoms returned. This suggests that diet was a major factor in both his disease progression and his recovery.

More recently, two new advocates of nutritional therapy for people with MS have emerged. Both are medical doctors, and both have MS themselves. Although the diets they are promoting are very different, they have both successfully treated themselves using diet, supplements and lifestyle changes.

Professor George Jelinek is a professor of emergency medicine who lives and works in Australia. He believes that lifestyle changes are the most effective therapies for chronic Western diseases such as MS, and in a quest to regain his health he developed the Overcoming MS diet. He advocates a plant-based wholefood diet with additional fish and seafood, plus either adequate sunlight or supplementation with vitamin D. He believes regular exercise and daily meditation are also essential.

Terry Wahls is an American doctor who started out using conventional drugs to treat her MS symptoms. However, they did not stop her disease progressing, and by the time she was regularly using a wheelchair she had begun to look for other options. As she researched the body's metabolism she came to believe that a version of the Palaeolithic or Stone Age diet was the answer, not only as a therapy for MS but as a way of fighting other autoimmune diseases such as rheumatoid arthritis and diabetes. Her diet is very high in nutrients and includes large amounts of organic vegetables and fruit each day, grass-fed meat and poultry and wild (not farmed) fish. It is also gluten-free and dairy-free and contains only small amount of grains and legumes. Dr Wahls no longer uses a wheelchair and she travels extensively promoting the diet, which she and her colleagues now use when treating patients with neurological diseases.

Why don't doctors advocate diet therapy?

As already noted, not many clinical trials have been carried out to monitor the effects of diet on people with MS. Such trials are normally funded by pharmaceutical companies, whose main aim is to sell drugs, not food. This makes it difficult to get financial backing for trials involving diet. Where trials have taken place, the results have often been disputed. Much of the evidence that diet works is anecdotal, and although some remarkable recoveries have been recorded, individual case studies – however impressive – are not enough to convince doctors, who have been trained to make decisions based on scientific evidence. The fact that most British medical schools include only very basic instruction in nutrition is also an obstacle.

In 1988, when I was diagnosed with MS, I was told that there is no evidence that diet has any effect on MS. This view was extremely common at the time. Indeed, there were (and maybe still are) some consultants who were actively hostile to the whole idea of diet therapy. The situation is slowly changing, and at least one UK university is now offering a postgraduate course in nutritional medicine. Nowadays many doctors – while not endorsing dietary changes – will not actively dissuade you from taking supplements such as fish oil or vitamin D. Some doctors believe there is now enough evidence in favour of dietary intervention to justify more clinical trials; indeed, a small scientific trial looking at the efficacy of the Best Bet diet took place in Scotland in 2007–8 (see page 59 for more details). However, until large-scale trials are carried out that successfully demonstrate how diet can help MS, medical professionals qualified to give you advice about how diet affects MS may continue to be thin on the ground.

The diets

Nutritional therapists agree that people with MS need to eat more of the 'right' foods and less of the 'wrong' foods, but there is less agreement on what exactly are the right and wrong foods. There are many types of diet that, over the years, have been claimed to benefit people with MS. Each type of diet has its advocates, and different diets will suit different people. In this book I have chosen to focus on five diets that, on the basis of research, anecdotal evidence and popularity, seem to offer the most potential benefits.

The healthy eating diet

The healthy eating diet is the sort of good basic diet that most doctors and dieticians would be happy to endorse, and not just for people with MS. It does not exclude any type of food completely but advises cutting down on fat, sugar, salt and refined foods and eating more fresh fruit and vegetables. Eating a healthy diet could do more than just help your MS symptoms. It should improve your general health and assist your body to fight off other illnesses. This is important because any illness, however minor, is an additional burden on your immune system. Your body's ability to cope with everyday ailments such as colds and flu is impaired if you get a fever, which can increase your core body temperature and exacerbate MS symptoms. People with MS may also take longer to recover from illness.

A healthy diet also helps protect you from other major diseases, such as cardiovascular disease, diabetes and some forms of cancer, and should help prevent weight gain, which can be a big problem if you cannot exercise effectively.

The healthy eating diet is the diet advocated by the MS Society of Great Britain. For a full description of the healthy eating diet and its vegetarian version, see Chapter 3.

The low-fat diet

The low-fat diet is based on the theory that fat intake is the crucial factor in the prevention and treatment of degenerative diseases, including multiple sclerosis. Bad (saturated) fats, which seem to be particularly harmful, are strictly limited, while consumption of beneficial fats in the form of unrefined oils, fish and supplements such as evening primrose oil is increased This diet is the one advocated by Professor Roy Swank, who was a pioneer in using diet as a therapy for MS. For full details of the low-fat diet see Chapter 4. I also include a description of a vegan diet, the vegetarian version of the low-fat diet.

The Best Bet diet

The Best Bet diet was pioneered by Dr Ashton Embry, a Canadian scientist. He believes that certain common proteins in foods such as dairy products and legumes must be excluded from the diet as they can trigger an immunological response that leads to MS. He also suggests MS can be helped by large therapeutic doses of vitamin D. A further component of the diet is identifying and eliminating food intolerances. You can find a description of the Best Bet diet in Chapter 5.

The Overcoming MS diet

The Overcoming MS diet is the diet promoted by Professor George Jelinek. This is basically a low-fat vegetarian diet with additional fish and seafood to provide omega-3 fats. Like the Best Bet diet, it excludes dairy products and limits sugar; however, gluten and legumes are allowed. Adequate vitamin D intake is also a feature, as well as regular exercise and daily meditation. For more details, see Chapter 6.

The Wahls diet

This is the diet advocated by Dr Terry Wahls in her book *The Wahls Protocol*. Dr Wahls believes that the key to treating MS and other immune diseases is feeding adequate nutrients to our mito-chondria, tiny organisms that provide the body with energy. Her diet is a variation of the Stone Age or Paleo diet. It eliminates all processed foods and replaces them with fresh organic vegetables, fruit, meat and poultry, line-caught fish and unrefined grains. Dairy products and gluten must also be avoided, and an adequate supply of vitamin D is essential. This is a high-fat, low-carbohy-drate diet, which in many ways runs contrary to current thinking on what constitutes a healthy diet and is quite complicated to follow. For this reason it is best carried out under medical supervi-sion. See Chapter 7 for more details.

Which diet?

Many people under 30 (the age group most likely to be diagnosed with MS) have never learnt the basics of nutrition or even been taught how to cook a simple meal. Their generation has grown up in a world where processed food, microwave meals and takeaways are the norm. Today, many people's food choices depend more on marketing, price and convenience than they do on health.

This wasn't always the case. In past times, patients were often sent to recuperate in the country, where good food, unpolluted air and adequate rest were also part of the therapeutic process.

If, like many people today, you regularly eat large quantities of unhealthy snacks, are addicted to fast food and often indulge in binge drinking, the healthy eating diet will show you a way of eating that is designed to prevent illness rather than encourage it. There is advice on how to plan a balanced diet, how to make healthy choices when shopping for food and how to cook simple and delicious dishes that promote good health. There are also recommendations for some basic supplements.

Those who feel better on the healthy eating diet but whose MS symptoms are still getting worse may see the low-fat diet as the next step. In this diet, fat intake is much more closely monitored. You will learn the difference between good fats and bad fats, how your body processes good fats and how to buy and use oils correctly so that they enhance your health rather than jeopardizing it. The low-fat vegetarian option – the vegan diet – is also explained, and advice is included on how to supplement with flaxseed oil and other essential fatty acids.

If you have failed to see an improvement on the low-fat diet or if your illness is progressing fast, you may decide that a more stringent diet such as the Overcoming MS diet or the Best Bet diet is what you need. For these more complicated diets where common foods such as dairy products or wheat are excluded, meal planning is essential, and you will probably find yourself doing more cooking than before, at least at first. If you are more than mildly disabled, you may need help with the cooking and shopping, at least until you have got the hang of the diet. Both the Best Bet diet and the Overcoming MS diet already have enthusiastic followers in the UK, Canada, the USA and Australia.

The Wahls diet is the most extreme of the diets and, as mentioned before, should preferably be undertaken under medical supervision. However, I have included details of this diet because some of its recommendations – such as eating a lot more vegetables each day – could benefit anyone with MS.

Unfortunately, there is no one diet that suits everybody with MS and, as with drugs, what works for one person will not necessarily work for another. When choosing which diet to follow, you need to consider such questions as cost (can I afford the cost of the sort of food and supplements recommended?), complexity (can I cope with the cooking and meal preparation that is required, either on my own or with help?) and preference (could I maintain this diet over the long term without getting fed up with it?). Before coming to a decision, it might be useful to discuss the options with your GP or MS nurse.

Above all, remember that these five diets are really just starters. Don't be afraid to adapt them to suit your own needs. Listen to what your body is telling you. If a food makes you feel bad, avoid it. If another food makes you feel good, eat more of it.

Food supplements

The orthodox medical view is that if you eat a healthy, balanced and varied diet you should get all the vitamins and minerals you need. Although this may be the case for the average healthy person in an ideal world, here are a few reasons why supplementation may be useful for someone with MS.

- It may not be possible, for all sorts of reasons, to stick to a healthy, balanced diet. Supplements should never be regarded as an acceptable alternative to a healthy diet, but they are a useful backup to ensure that if your diet lapses you won't go short of essential nutrients.
- Much of the processed and refined food available today is deficient in nutrients.
- Pesticide residues on fruit and vegetables may prevent absorption of nutrients.
- Food contains its optimum level of nutrients when it is fresh. Vitamins and minerals are lost during storage and again in the cooking process.
- Some people with MS may have difficulty absorbing nutrients. Moreover, they may need a larger dose because of their illness.
- Taking the contraceptive pill, drinking alcohol and smoking are just some of the things that can deplete the body of vital nutrients.

- If your diet prevents you from eating certain categories of food (if you are a vegan or your diet excludes gluten or dairy products, for example), you may need to take extra vitamins and minerals to replace those in the foods you no longer eat.

Supplements that can help MS

Vitamin B complex

The B complex vitamins are important for the functioning of the brain and nerves and for a healthy digestive system. Because they all work together, they are often prescribed in the form of a single B complex supplement.

B vitamins that are particularly important for MS include B_1, which helps improve memory, muscle strength and fatigue, and B_6, which is vital for the health of both the nervous and immune systems and the production of the hormone serotonin, which controls our mood. In addition, B_3, B_6 and biotin are needed to convert EFAs into the more complex fatty acids and eventually into prostaglandins (see pages 49–50). Trials are currently taking place in France to see if high-dose biotin could have a therapeutic effect on progressive MS.

Many people with MS appear to be deficient in vitamin B_{12}, which plays a crucial role in the formation of myelin. B_{12} is not assimilated well by the gut, so it is quite common for it to be given in the form of an injection. Vitamin B_{12} can help a range of MS symptoms such as fatigue, pins and needles and depression. It is possible to have a blood test to check the levels of B_{12} in your blood, but such tests are not always conclusive. B_{12} is only available from animal sources. This leaves vegetarians and vegans at particular risk of deficiency.

- **Food sources of B vitamins** Whole grains, dairy foods, meat, oily fish, eggs, nuts and dark-green leafy vegetables.
- **Food sources of vitamin B_{12}** Offal, red meat, oily fish, white fish and dairy products.

Antioxidants

Antioxidants, which include vitamins A, C and E and the mineral selenium, combat damage caused by free radicals, tiny electrons that help to oxidate the body and kill bacteria. Sometimes, however, they become too numerous and start to damage the body. Free radical damage is thought to be a factor in MS. Antioxidants also help to decrease the fragility of blood capillaries, which may help prevent the breakdown of the blood–brain barrier.

Vitamin A is very important for the health of the eyes, while vitamin C plays a part in the EFA conversion process and also helps strengthen the immune system against infection. Vitamin E works in conjunction with selenium to boost immunity and also helps blood circulation. Some recent studies have shown an increased death rate among people taking vitamins A and E in the form of a supplement, so it may be wise to obtain these antioxidants from a dietary source.

- **Food sources for antioxidants** See pages 36–7.

Vitamin D

To see why adequate vitamin D intake is an important part of several of the diets featured in this book, you need to understand how vitamin D affects the body. The sun's ultraviolet rays produce vitamin D, which is then transformed into a substance known as circulating vitamin D. This is transported round the body via the blood and used by cells to produce the vitamin D hormone. Immune cells in particular need adequate vitamin D hormone to regulate the immune system and prevent damage to the body's own tissues (autoimmune disease).

It has now been established that people living in sunny climates where MS is rare have a level of circulating vitamin D of 100–150 nmol/L (nanomols per litre).This level also protects against osteoporosis. Professor Jelinek recommends that people with MS should be aiming for a blood level above 150 nmol/L, while their close relatives should aim for levels above 100 nmol/L to prevent them from developing MS themselves.

Research into the links between vitamin D deficiency and MS is continuing, and now scientists at McGill University in Canada have found strong evidence of a causal link between lack of vitamin D and susceptibility to MS. Their research seems to validate the suggestion that vitamin D is one of the environmental factors that plays a part in the development of MS. More recently still, a team at the University of Cambridge have been investigating the possible use of vitamin D in myelin repair. They found that by adding vitamin D to proteins in brain cells, the production rate of myelin-creating cells increased by 80 per cent. This work seems to support the importance of an adequate supply of vitamin D for people with MS.

Vitamin D deficiency is now also being implicated in many other chronic medical conditions including osteoporosis, cardiovascular disease, rheumatoid arthritis and diabetes.

So what is the best way to obtain your daily dose of vitamin D? Getting enough vitamin D from diet alone is not really an option, as you would need to eat at least two portions of oily fish a day. If you live in a country where the sun shines all year round, you should try to get at least 15 minutes of sun exposure every day onto as much of your body as possible, with a bit more on days when the sun is less strong. If this is not possible, then you will need to take supplements.

Vitamin D_3 is preferable to D_2, which has to be converted to D_3 in the body. Vitamin D is fat-soluble, so it is best taken in capsule form as the oil in the capsule helps the active ingredient to be absorbed into the body. If you take it as a pill, it should be eaten with some form of fatty food. Vitamin D is also available as drops or a mouth spray, which could be useful if you have problems swallowing.

Your GP can arrange for you to have a 25 (OH)D blood test to establish your nmol/L levels. Although the current recommended daily allowance (RDA) for vitamin D is 400 iu, there is growing evidence that this is much too low. Recent research in Iran has established that you can safely take up to 7,000 iu per day or 50,000 iu per week to boost the vitamin D in your body to the desired level. Some health professionals recommend a mega-dose to start with, followed by a much lower maintenance dose. Your GP or MS nurse will be able to advise you on dosages.

- **Food sources of vitamin D** Oily fish, eggs, liver.

Calcium

This is needed for myelin synthesis. It is also essential for the health of teeth and bones, and our need for it grows with age. Poor absorption of food due to food intolerances or leaky gut can give rise to a calcium deficiency, and if you omit dairy foods from your diet you will almost certainly need to take a supplement. Adequate vitamin D, magnesium and vitamin K_2 are also needed for calcium utilization, and these nutrients, working together, can help prevent osteoporosis.

- **Food sources of calcium** Tofu, dairy products, tinned sardines and salmon, dark-green leafy vegetables, cauliflower, nuts and seeds, dried apricots and figs.

Magnesium

Magnesium works closely with calcium to facilitate the transmission of nerve impulses to muscles. Like zinc, it is also important in the conversion of EFAs. Deficiency can cause muscle spasms and incontinence.

- **Food sources of magnesium** Soya beans, nuts, whole grains, meat, eggs, bananas and dark-green leafy vegetables.

Iron

Iron is essential for the production of haemoglobin, which transports oxygen and carbon dioxide around the body and is important for energy production in cells. Since the best sources of iron are animal products, vegetarians and vegans are at particular risk of iron deficiency (anaemia), as are menstruating women and the elderly. Anaemia can cause fatigue and impaired immunity, so anyone with MS would be well advised to ask their GP to test their iron levels and, if necessary, prescribe a supplement.

- **Food sources of iron** Shellfish, red meat, sardines, egg yolks, wheatgerm, green vegetables, quinoa and dried fruit. Note that iron from plant sources is less well absorbed by the body than iron from animal sources.

Zinc

Zinc teams up with vitamin B in conversion of EFAs and, like vitamin C, it helps to protect the body against infection. Zinc deficiency is very common in people with MS and may be a reason why they sometimes lose their sense of taste. The older you are, the more likely you are to be deficient in zinc.

To test for zinc deficiency, you can buy a solution of zinc sulphate from a chemist. Swill a teaspoonful round your mouth. If you can't taste anything, you are almost certainly deficient in zinc.

- **Food sources of zinc** Red meat, seafood, liver, whole grains, pulses, eggs, almonds and Brazil nuts, pumpkin seeds.

Other minerals

Other minerals such as copper, selenium and manganese may also be beneficial to people with MS. The easiest way to take these is as a multimineral supplement, but therapists may recommend larger doses of a particular mineral if they feel you may be deficient in it.

EFAs

A description of the different types of EFAs and their importance to health can be found in Chapter 4 on the low-fat diet.

Probiotics

Probiotics such as lactobaccillus and bifidobacterium are organisms that live in the gut. Our stomachs contain trillions of bacteria and, ideally, 70 per cent of these should be good (probiotic) bacteria, as they help to discourage the other 30 per cent, which are harmful, from proliferating. Unfortunately, some drugs, such as steroids and antibiotics, kill off the good bacteria, so sometimes you may need to take a probiotic supplement to help rebalance your gut flora.

- **Food sources of probiotics** Live yogurt, fermented milk drinks.

Choosing supplements

Organic supplements are preferable to inorganic supplements as they may have a higher absorption rate. They often come in capsule form, which means they are likely to contain fewer additional substances, such as binding agents, and more of the active ingredient.

Always buy the best quality supplements you can afford from a reputable supplier, one who can provide you with technical information and answer any queries you have. Cheap supplements may contain only small quantities of the active ingredient, or the ingredient itself may be of poor quality. They are unlikely to deliver the therapeutic benefits you need.

Choosing probiotics

Each probiotic should contain a minimum of 4,000,000 live bacteria. The most beneficial strains are *Lactobacillus acidophilus* and bifidobacterium. Unfortunately, some products may not contain as many bacteria as they claim or they may contain additional undesirable bacteria or the sort that is unable to survive stomach acid. A reputable manufacturer should be able to give you full technical information including the correct dosage and whether to take them with food or between meals.

Buy capsules, not tablets, as the manufacturing process for tablets compromises the product's viability. Probiotics are available in powder form for those who cannot swallow capsules. Some probiotics are manufactured using a fermentation process that involves milk, but it is possible to buy milk-free probiotics if you need to avoid cow's milk. Before you buy, check the expiry date and whether or not the product needs to be refrigerated.

The correct dosage

RDAs are guidelines suggesting how much of each vitamin and mineral we need each day in order to stay healthy. Experts in nutrition believe that different individuals have different nutritional needs according to their age and their state of health. There is therefore no 'right' or 'wrong' level of dosage for everyone. This is why it is helpful to get advice from a qualified practitioner to ensure you are taking the correct amount of a supplement for your particular needs.

People who are ill often need larger doses of nutrients than healthy people (therapeutic doses). There is, however, a maximum safe dose for each nutrient and taking more than this can be dangerous. For more detailed information see Dr Sarah Brewer, *The Essential Guide to Vitamins, Minerals and Herbal Supplements*, or look at the Health Supplements Information Service website (<www.hsis.org>).

Here are a few safety guidelines.

- Remember that different brands of the same supplement may come in different strengths. Follow the manufacturer's instructions for dosage or consult a nutritional therapist who can confirm the correct dosage for you.
- If you are already taking a prescription drug, check with your

doctor or pharmacist before you start taking any supplements. Some vitamins, minerals and herbal supplements can interact with drugs and cause problems.

- If you need an operation, it is important that both your consultant and the hospital anaesthetist know which supplements and/or herbal medicines you are taking. You may need to stop taking them before the operation.
- Some nutrients – such as vitamin A – should not be taken in large doses while pregnant or breastfeeding. There are some, however – such as folic acid – that are positively beneficial when you are pregnant as they may help to prevent foetal abnormalities. Either way, it is best to get advice from a qualified therapist on which supplements to take and which to avoid in this situation.
- Take supplements with food or within 20 minutes of a meal. Fat-soluble substances, such as vitamins A, D and E, should be taken with food containing fat, such as milk. Take all other supplements with either water or orange juice, not tea or coffee, which may prevent their absorption.

2

Other factors to consider

Food intolerance

Testing for possible food intolerances and then eliminating suspect foods is part of the Best Bet diet. Why is this? Let's start by defining the difference between food intolerance and food allergy. A food allergy is a reaction (usually immediate) to eating a particular food. A severe reaction can cause the body to go into anaphylactic shock, a life-threatening condition. The offending substance can be pinpointed by a skin-prick or RAST test, which indicates if antibodies are present in the blood. It must then be avoided completely to prevent future reactions. Very often, it is foods that are eaten less frequently that are the culprits, such as nuts or prawns.

With food intolerance, on the other hand, the symptoms are less severe than in an allergic reaction but can be a lot more insidious. Foods that cause intolerance tend to be the ones – such as wheat and milk – that we eat in large quantities on a regular basis, so that the effect is sometimes masked. They are also often the foods that we crave the most. Food intolerances do not usually show up on skin-prick or RAST tests and often go undetected, sometimes for years. Moreover, many doctors in the UK, while acknowledging that there is such a thing as food intolerance, believe that it is fairly rare.

Unfortunately, few trials involving food sensitivity have been carried out in this country, and there is controversy over the findings of most of those that have. Until more scientific evidence is available, doctors may continue to underestimate this problem.

Food intolerance and MS

Food intolerance can have a direct effect on the body's ability to assimilate nutrients; it can affect the way the digestive organs function and, in particular, may prevent the body breaking down fat properly. Dr Embry, instigator of the Best Bet diet, believes food intolerances may be responsible for the breaching of the blood–brain barrier, which may be one factor involved in the onset of MS. Different foods affect different people in different ways. This is one of the reasons it's so difficult to carry out controlled tests involving food sensitivities. It also means it's impossible to predict which of your symptoms might improve once you give up a certain food. All you can do is omit the suspect food and see what happens. Chronic fatigue, depression, muscle and joint pains, diarrhoea and constipation, headaches and food cravings are just some of the symptoms that can be indicative of food intolerance.

Finding out if you have food intolerances

There are several options.

Elimination diet

The only medically approved and scientifically proven method of identifying food intolerances is to go on an elimination diet and then slowly reintroduce suspect foods one by one to see if they cause a reaction. This is probably the most reliable method of diagnosing food intolerances if carried out correctly, and it is the method used in NHS allergy clinics. If you suffer from hay fever, asthma, eczema or allergic rhinitis (constant runny nose) you could ask for a referral to one of these clinics, but having MS would not normally be considered an adequate reason for such a referral.

The most common allergens are wheat, milk, egg, citrus fruit, yeast, chocolate and additives. If you do have food sensitivities, you are likely to see a reduction in symptoms within seven to ten days, and reintroduction of the culprit foods will then trigger a recurrence of symptoms.

It is possible to carry out this process yourself. For a step-by-step guide, see *The Complete Guide to Food Allergy and Intolerance* by Professor Jonathan Brostoff and Linda Gamlin, which explains the different options open to you. To carry out an elimination diet effectively, you need to stick to the diet faithfully for the required length of time or the results will not be reliable.

Warning If you have ever had a severe reaction to a food in the past or you suffered from atopic eczema as a child, you should not attempt the elimination and reintroduction of suspect foods without medical support or you could risk going into anaphylactic shock when you reintroduce a culprit food.

Food diary

The charity Allergy UK suggests keeping a record for a couple of months of everything you consume – food, drink, medication, supplements – and any symptoms you experience. Correlating food and symptoms may give you some ideas about what it is you are sensitive to. Food diaries can sometimes produce unexpected results. For instance, I found out by using a food diary that whenever I took evening primrose oil I would get severe muscle spasms. You can be sensitive to anything, even foods generally regarded as beneficial.

Blood tests

Blood tests designed to detect food intolerances, such as the ELISA blood test recommended by the Best Bet diet group, are known as IgG tests. Everybody makes IgG antibodies to food, and the testers claim that a person with a food intolerance will make more IgG antibodies than a healthy person would. Unfortunately, factors such as how often you eat a food or whether you have a 'leaky gut' can cause IgG levels in blood to vary, and this can compromise the accuracy of the test. This, together with the fact that little research has been done into the relationship between IgG antibodies and food intolerance, is why most doctors do not endorse these tests. If you do decide to go down this route, the ELISA blood test is available from Cambridge Nutritional Sciences in the UK (see page 146 for details).

'Alternative' methods

Many complementary health clinics offer 'alternative' methods of testing for food intolerances, such as Vega tests, applied kinesiology and pulse rate changes. There is no scientific proof that any of these methods work, so if you are considering using one of these clinics, proceed cautiously. Check what testing methods they use, what qualifications the staff have, and what their success rate is in accurately pinpointing food sensitivities. This is important, because if you are already omitting some categories of food from your diet, the last thing you need is to be told to omit foods that actually do you no harm.

Can I combine nutritional medicine with drug therapy?

If you are receiving disease-modifying drugs such as Betaferon or Copaxone, you can still modify your diet and get the resultant health benefits. You don't have to choose between the two approaches. It is important, though, to let your GP or neurologist know what supplements you are taking, as some combinations of drugs and supplements can cause harm.

Are these diets suitable for anyone with MS?

There are a few points to bear in mind before you start to follow one of the diets in this book.

If you are already following another special diet for medical reasons (because you are diabetic, for example), you should always discuss any proposed changes with a dietician or your local MS nurse or GP before you start. The same advice applies if you are pregnant, breastfeeding or trying to conceive.

Whatever foods you exclude from your diet, make sure you eat enough protein. This is very important in order to maintain your energy levels. The protein can come from animal or vegetable sources, depending on which diet you are following, but aim to consume about 350 g (12 oz) of protein per day. It is not possible to follow the Best Bet diet if you are a vegetarian or vegan, because omitting dairy products, legumes and pulses will leave you short of protein.

If you decide to omit a food or a group of foods, replace it either with another food that contains the same nutrients or with an appropriate supplement.

Don't go on any form of exclusion diet if you are seriously underweight or if you suffer from an eating disorder. In these circumstances the healthy eating diet is as far as you should go.

Swallowing problems

Some people with MS have trouble swallowing food and liquid (dysphagia). This is a problem that often affects those with more advanced MS, but it can also be experienced by people with less severe forms of the disease. Symptoms can include problems with chewing and swallowing; food particles sticking in the throat, sometimes leading to choking; and excessive saliva.

There are several risks associated with this condition. Instead of passing down the oesophagus, food and liquid may trickle into the airways and eventually reach the lungs, with a risk of causing respiratory infections. People may also eat and drink less than they would normally because they are anxious about potential problems such as choking, and this may lead to them becoming malnourished or dehydrated.

There are things you can do to help yourself if you suffer from dysphagia.

- Eat and drink in a relaxed atmosphere and allow yourself plenty of time to eat your meal.
- Sit upright and tuck your chin in as you swallow. This helps to close airways, making choking less likely.
- Take small mouthfuls and sips of liquid and chew each mouthful well before you swallow it.
- Don't try to talk while eating.
- Cold liquids or hot, thickened liquids, such as soups or tea with milk, are easier to swallow than hot thin liquids, such as herbal tea.
- Moist, soft foods are easier to swallow, so purée or liquefy foods before eating. Alternatively, add a thick liquid, such as gravy or custard, to drier foods.
- Alternate liquid and solid food.
- At the end of the meal, drink a small amount of liquid and cough once or twice to dislodge any remaining particles. Sit upright for 30 minutes after you have finished eating to help the digestive process.

Many of the recipes in this book would be suitable for people with swallowing problems, such as smoothies; porridge; pasta dishes (so long as the meat, fish and vegetables are in small pieces and well softened in the cooking process, such as Sardine Pasta, see page 114); puréed soups such as sweet potato and coriander; and desserts such as Apricot and Banana Granola Crumble and Apple Snow (pages 128 and 127).

If you want to take supplements and you cannot swallow conventional tablets or capsules, some vitamins and minerals, such as vitamin C, are now available in powder form and can be dissolved in liquid for easier consumption.

If you have been diagnosed with dysphagia, you are likely to be referred to a dietician and you should discuss any potential dietary changes with him or her.

How long will it take for a change in diet to bring health benefits?

Our bodies are regenerating themselves all the time. Wounds heal; broken bones knit together; cut hair regrows. It takes about two years for the entire human body to be rebuilt. Depending on how severe and longstanding your symptoms are, it could take at least this time for all possible improvements to take place. Anecdotal evidence suggests that people who start to use diet therapy as soon as they are diagnosed sometimes see very quick improvements, while those who have been ill for several years may have to wait much longer in order to get results. However, if you have seen no improvement in your health after six months, or if some of your symptoms are worse, you should reconsider whether this is the right diet for you. Bear in mind too that with a disease such as MS there is a point of no return, after which some damage may be irreversible. Once you have received a firm diagnosis, the sooner you start the dietary approach the better, in order to obtain the best possible outcome.

Diet and other conditions

Developing additional autoimmune diseases is always a possibility when the immune system is not functioning properly. In fact, while researching this book I was surprised to discover how many people with MS have also been diagnosed with other illnesses such as coeliac disease, Hughes Syndrome, rheumatoid arthritis or Type 1 diabetes.

For coeliac disease, dietary intervention is a medically approved treatment; coeliacs have to stick to a gluten-free diet for life. Diabetes, too, involves a medically approved diet that is very similar to the healthy eating diet in that it recommends regular intake of unrefined starchy foods to control blood sugar levels, a reduction in fat, sugar and salt and an increased consumption of fruit, vegetables and oily fish. There is also evidence that eating less saturated fat and more fish oil, and identifying food sensitivities, is helpful in healing rheumatoid arthritis.

In all immune diseases the immune system, instead of protecting the body from attack, itself attacks parts of the body it sees as a threat. Dr Terry Wahls, in *The Wahls Protocol*, states that all immune diseases share a further five characteristics:

1 mitochondria produce energy less efficiently, leading to excess production of free radicals;
2 inflammation occurs throughout the body;
3 toxins and chronic infections worsen symptoms;
4 vitamin D levels are low and stress hormone levels high;
5 the body is deficient in vitamins, minerals and EFAs.

Dr Wahls suggests that faulty biochemistry is the cause of all auto-immune diseases, including MS, and that therefore detoxing the body and providing it with all the nutrients it needs is crucial in the healing process.

Protecting your family

Multiple sclerosis isn't hereditary, but the children of a man or woman with MS have a 1 in 48 chance of contracting it, so they are theoretically more at risk than the general population, whose chances of getting MS are 1 in 330.

Genes, however, make up only half the risk factors in whether or not you get MS; the other risk factors are environmental. We do not yet know for sure whether diet is one of these risk factors, but it makes sense to help protect your children's health by encouraging them to eat a healthy diet and teaching them how to cook nutritious meals, especially since studies in the USA and Sweden have found that young people who are overweight at 20 are at greater risk of developing MS in later life.

It is also important for those who care for people with MS to eat a healthy diet themselves. Caring can be stressful, and stress can make you ill. When you are exhausted from looking after someone else's needs, it is all too easy to neglect your own.

Dr Ashton Embry, pioneer of the Best Bet diet, suggests that lack of vitamin D may be a trigger for MS in people who are genetically vulnerable (that is, people with a family history of MS). He believes that we can help protect young people, particularly those who live in cooler climates such as Britain and Canada, by giving them vitamin D supplements from an early age. This seems good advice when you consider how many children today spend hours in darkened rooms playing computer games rather than running around out of doors. For more guidance on vitamin D supplementation for children, consult your GP or MS nurse.

Part 2
THE DIETS

3

The healthy eating diet

Many people are confused about exactly what constitutes a healthy diet. However, there is broad agreement among members of the medical professions, dieticians and nutritionists on what we should be eating to promote health and well-being, and what we should cut down on if we don't want to become ill. If you follow the seven principles below, you won't go far wrong.

1 Eat less saturated fat

Saturated fats are bad for us in several ways.

They can form sticky platelets that clump together and clog up arteries, leading to the formation of blood clots and strokes.

Saturated fats increase the amount of cholesterol in the bloodstream. Cholesterol is one factor in atherosclerosis, where deposits of protein, fats, cholesterol and minerals narrow arteries, cutting off blood supplies and nutrients to the organs they serve. Blocked arteries can cause stroke, heart attack, pulmonary embolism or gangrene. Cholesterol cannot easily be broken down by the body; it has to be excreted and this requires an adequate fibre intake. This is why a diet full of saturated fat (fried food and red meat) and low in fibre (fruit and vegetables) is so bad for health.

Atherosclerosis also hardens arteries, making them less resilient, and this in turn raises blood pressure, another factor in heart disease. There is also evidence that a high-fat diet is particularly bad for people with MS (see the low-fat diet, Chapter 4).

Fats that are hard at room temperature, such as lard, butter and suet, are called saturated fats. Red meat (beef, pork and lamb) often contains a lot of saturated fat, and so do some types of poultry such as duck and geese, although chicken and turkey are low-fat meats apart from the skin. Processed foods such as pies, sausages, pâtés, chocolate, cakes and biscuits are all likely to be high in saturated fat, as are crisps and chips and any food that has been fried.

Ways to cut down on saturated fats

- Buy lean cuts of meat and cut off visible fat before cooking.
- Use a rack in the roasting tray or grill pan when cooking meat or chicken so that excess fat can drain away.
- Eat less fried food and fry in oil rather than butter or lard. Use the smallest possible amount of oil required to prevent food from sticking to the pan. Never reuse cooking oil.
- Try to avoid deep-fried food such as chips altogether. Instead, choose low-fat varieties of oven chips.
- Replace butter with polyunsaturated margarine on bread and toast, and use olive oil in cooking.
- Limit yourself to four medium eggs a week (unless you are underweight).

2 Eat fewer refined carbohydrates

Carbohydrates (starches and sugars) fuel the body's energy systems and metabolism and are our main source of calories. Our ancestors ate a lot of complex carbohydrates, found in fruit, vegetables, pulses and whole grains. The modern Western diet, on the other hand, contains far more refined carbohydrates in the form of white flour, white rice and white sugar. These foods have been heavily processed in ways that destroy much of their natural goodness. They contain only 'empty' calories that make you fat while at the same time leaving you short of vitamins, minerals and dietary fibre. Eat too many of these foods and you could suffer from malnutrition even while being overweight. If you have MS it is particularly important to avoid foods that will encourage weight gain without giving you any health benefit.

Refined carbohydrates are predigested so they bypass our digestive systems and give us a quick burst of energy. However, this type of energy won't last long. Complex carbohydrates, on the other hand, release energy more slowly over a longer period and also provide essential nutrients.

Sugar has the potential to cause more damage than any other refined carbohydrate, triggering conditions such as diabetes and hyperglycaemia, which can make your blood sugar levels fluctuate wildly and cause sugar cravings. Sugar can give you a quick energy boost, but when your levels fall again you crave more sweet food.

Sugary drinks are a particular problem. A recent survey by Action on Sugar tested the sugar content of canned fizzy drinks. Of the cans tested, 79 per cent contained at least 6 teaspoonfuls of sugar: colas contained 9, while some ginger beers contained 13! You can make your own healthy fizzy drinks from a small amount of fruit juice mixed with sparkling spring water.

The World Health Organization currently recommends that sugars should form no more than 10 per cent of our daily calorie intake, but it is considering reducing this target further to 5 per cent.

Research at the University of Alabama has shown that white sugar has a rapid and adverse effect upon the ability of white blood cells to fight infection. This suggests that people who have recurrent infections or infections that don't respond to normal treatment should consider avoiding white sugar completely.

Simply using artificial sweeteners instead of sugar isn't the answer either, as they just encourage your sweet tooth. Why not start by replacing your usual sugary snacks with fresh or dried fruit or fruit smoothies (see page 94) and using natural sweeteners such as honey, maple syrup or muscovado (the least refined form of sugar) instead of white sugar.

Good carbs – eat more of these

- Wholemeal and granary bread and rolls.
- Wholegrain cereals, such as Shredded Wheat and Weetabix.
- Oats in the form of porridge (but not the quick-cook variety), muesli or oatcakes.
- Pasta made from unrefined flours, such as brown rice, buckwheat or maize.
- Brown rice or other unrefined whole grains, such as millet or quinoa.
- Wholegrain crackers, such as Ryvita.
- Starchy vegetables, such as sweetcorn, broccoli and cauliflower. Note that potatoes, though starchy, should not be eaten in large quantities as they tend to break down quickly in the body like refined carbohydrates.

Bad carbs – eat less of these

- White bread and rolls.
- Refined, sugary cereals and sugary drinks such as cola.

- All forms of refined rice and pasta.
- Cakes, pastries, biscuits, crackers, confectionery and other manu-factured goodies made with white flour and white sugar.

3 Eat more fish

Fish, especially oily fish such as tuna, mackerel and salmon, is full of omega-3 essential fatty acids. These can't be made by the body; you can only get them by eating the right foods. The additional importance of EFAs to people with MS is explained in Chapter 4, but there are many other good reasons for eating fish.

- Fish is a good source of low-fat protein.
- It's quick and easy to cook and delicious to eat.
- Oily fish such as salmon and trout contain vitamin D, which is a crucial nutrient for people with MS.
- Tinned oily fish with bones, such as sardines, are an excellent source of calcium.
- White fish is a good source of the antioxidant selenium, which is often missing in the modern diet.
- Shellfish are another good source of low-fat protein. However, they are also a source of cholesterol so if you have high blood pressure or a heart condition it may be better to avoid them.

4 Eat low-fat dairy products

Dairy products are good protein foods and useful sources of calcium (although by no means the only ones). However, most of them, such as cream, cream cheese, hard cheeses such as Cheddar and ice-cream, are naturally high in saturated fat. Cut down on these foods and eat more low-fat dairy products, such as:

- skimmed or semi-skimmed milk
- low-fat natural yogurt (but not the flavoured, low-fat yogurts as extra sugar may have been added to compensate for the lack of fat)
- fromage frais – virtually fat-free (0.4 per cent fat) or creamy (7.9 per cent fat)
- cottage cheese or curd cheese
- quark – a soft white cheese made from fermented skimmed milk that is virtually fat-free; a useful ingredient in dips
- half-fat Cheddar.

5 Eat five portions of fruit and vegetables daily

The World Health Organization recommends that we all eat at least five portions of fruit and vegetables every day in order to stay healthy. Recent research suggests that upping your intake to seven portions a day could cut even further your risk of dying from cancer or heart disease.

Fresh fruit and vegetables are best because they contain most nutrients, but frozen, tinned and dried varieties also count towards your five portions a day, as do pulses (peas, beans and lentils). If you have a glass of fruit juice with your breakfast, a salad at lunch, a portion of cooked vegetables with your evening meal and a couple of pieces of fruit between meals, you'll easily achieve your five a day.

Smoothies are another delicious way of eating fruit (see page 94) and you can use raw celery sticks, carrot or cucumber as dippers with dishes such as hummus (see page 100). In hot weather you can also pour fruit juice, puréed fruit or fruit smoothies into lolly moulds and freeze them – a really delicious way of cooling down!

Tubs of rice or pasta salad are good lunch-box fillers, and adding slices of tomato, cucumber and pepper to sandwiches makes them taste more interesting as well as bumping up their nutritional value.

It is particularly important if you have MS to eat a helping of dark-green leafy vegetables, such as cabbage, spinach, broccoli or greens, every day, as they contain large quantities of magnesium, which will help oxygenate your blood and also help prevent all sorts of problems such as constipation, depression and tired-ness. Don't overcook vegetables as this destroys the nutrients (see instructions for preparing and cooking vegetables on pages 102–5). Don't leave fruit and vegetables lying around too long before you eat them, as they lose nutrients with each passing day.

So what exactly is a 'portion' of fruit and vegetables? Here are some guidelines:

- 1 medium-sized piece of fruit, such as an apple, banana or orange
- 10–15 cherries or grapes
- 2 smaller fruits, such as plums or satsumas
- 1 tablespoon of dried fruit, such as raisins
- 1 slice of melon
- 1 glass 100 per cent pure fruit juice
- 1 tomato, 1 onion or half a pepper

Table 3.1 Fruit and vegetables in season

Try to buy fruit and vegetables in season when they are at their tasty, succulent best. Produce that has been flown in from abroad out of season is more expensive and will almost certainly have lost some of its nutrient content.

Fruit	In season
Apples (English)	September to November
Apricots	June to August
Cherries	June, July
Figs	September
Grapes	December to March
Grapefruit	December to March
Nuts	October to December
Oranges	January to March
Peaches	June to September
Pears	September to February
Plums	August
Raspberries	July, August
Rhubarb	December to June
Strawberries	May to July
Tangerines	December

Vegetables	In Season
Asparagus	May, June
Aubergine	June to August
Beans (green)	May to September
Beetroot	July to April
Broccoli	June to November
Brussels sprouts	August to March
Cauliflower	July to April
Celery	June to August
Celeriac	December to May
Corn on the cob	July to September
Courgettes	May to October
Fennel	June to August
Garlic	September to November
Leek	December to May
Lettuce	May to October
New potatoes	April to June
Parsnips	September to April
Peppers	May to September
Radishes	April to June
Spinach	March, April
Tomatoes	June to November
Watercress	March to August

NB: Onions, carrots, cabbages, mushrooms and salad cress are available all year round.

- 1 heaped tablespoon of carrots, peas or sweetcorn
- 1 cereal bowlful of salad.

Note that you can only count juice as one portion, however much you drink in one day, and potatoes don't count towards your five a day because they are classified as a carbohydrate.

Table 3.1 lists when fruit and vegetables are in season.

6 Eat less salt

The RDA for salt for an adult is 6 g (1 tsp). However, as 75 per cent of the salt we eat is already in the food we buy, such as bread and cereals, you may not be aware of how much you are eating.

A recent study in Argentina that investigated the link between salt intake and MS symptoms found that those participants who consumed a large amount of salt in their diet had a measureable increase in disease activity.

According to scientists at the University of Vermont, salt may also turn out to be one of the environmental factors contributing to MS, as their research suggests that salt has an influence on the immune cells that cause MS.

Both these studies suggest that you would be wise to cut down on salty foods, such as crisps, and look for low-salt options when buying processed foods.

Salt clogs up the arteries and can be a contributory factor in heart disease, so cutting your intake will also benefit your general health. Try substituting black pepper and herbs and spices for salt in recipes to enhance flavour.

7 Ensure you drink enough liquid

Our bodies need water to help absorb nutrients and to flush out toxins and waste matter. Few of us drink enough liquid, and this can lead to problems as varied as headaches, mood changes and constipation.

Try to drink six to eight glasses of liquid per day, preferably in the form of water, herb tea or diluted fruit juice rather than tea, coffee and alcohol, which act as diuretics and flush essential minerals from the body. People who are very active may need more.

Don't make the mistake of drinking less in order to minimize visits to the toilet. Your urine will become concentrated, which can irritate your bladder and encourage bladder infections. If you are prone to these, why not drink a large glass of cranberry juice every day? Finnish researchers have found that tannins in the juice have an antibacterial effect, which helps prevent bladder infections.

It's easy to become dehydrated. If you're busy, you may forget to drink, or you may confuse thirst with hunger and eat instead of drinking. Urine that is dark yellow instead of clear and pale is a sign that you are not drinking enough liquid.

If you drink filtered water, remember that the filter will remove beneficial minerals as well as harmful chemicals, so it is advisable to take a multimineral supplement. Make sure you change the filter as often as the manufacturer recommends, or you could become ill. Carbonated water has the same effect, as the carbon minerals bind to the other minerals in the water and remove them from your body. Naturally sparkling spring water is a better bet.

A useful product for anyone who has a problem transporting, holding or lifting drinks is the Hydrant, which clips on to a belt, bed or wheelchair and has a flexible plastic drinking tube (see page 147 for purchase details).

Superfoods

Most health professionals agree that foods containing antioxidants are extremely beneficial. (The reasons for this are given on page 13.) Here are some of the most useful antioxidant-rich foods.

- **Blueberries** Dark berries, such as blueberries, blackberries and blackcurrants, contain some of the most powerful natural anti-oxidants in existence. Blueberries and cranberries also contain a compound that helps prevent bacteria sticking to the lining of the bladder so they can protect against cystitis and bladder infections.
- **Tomatoes** Tomatoes contain high levels of vitamin C. Heating them releases an antioxidant called lycopene, which has anti-cancer properties, and cooking them with olive oil increases absorption of the lycopene. Lycopene is also found in red peppers and watermelons.
- **Carrots** Carrots are a good source of carotene, which converts into vitamin A in the body and helps reduce your risk of heart disease and cancer. Regular intakes can help reduce cholesterol levels and prevent macular degeneration and cataracts, which can lead to blindness. Carrots also contain vitamin C, potas-

sium, calcium, iron and zinc. Eat them with a little oil or fat to encourage absorption of the carotene.

- **Dark-green leafy vegetables** Spring greens, spinach, kale, chard and broccoli are all good sources of vitamins C and E and carotenoids. They are also rich in calcium, potassium (which helps prevent calcium loss) and folic acid and are a good source of fibre. Broccoli has been shown to have anti-cancer properties. It contains lipoic acid, which has been linked with increased brain power and energy, and lutein, which helps maintain healthy eyes. Broccoli and spinach both also contain co-enzyme Q10, which is needed for cellular energy.

- **Green tea** All tea is rich in antioxidants, but green tea also has anti-inflammatory and neuro-protective qualities that particularly benefit people with MS. In addition, it kills the streptococcus bacteria that encourage tooth decay and gum disease. Use four tea bags to one mug of hot water and steep for 10 minutes for full therapeutic benefit. Green tea contains caffeine, but the herbal extract (available at health food shops) does not.

Organic or not?

While only approved pesticides and chemicals can be used in the production of fruit and vegetables on commercial farms, some chemicals that are banned from food production in other countries are deemed safe in the UK. Alternatively, some substances banned in the UK are still used on imported produce. Until we have international agreement on what is safe and what is not, we cannot be sure what we are eating. Recently, 174 scientists from 28 countries jointly participated in a project to investigate the 'cocktail effect' of mixing different approved chemicals in the food we eat. They concluded that one in five cancers may be caused when chemicals deemed safe on their own blend lethally inside the human body.

Official data shows that over the past 50 years there has been a steady decline in mineral levels in fruit and vegetables. Nutrient levels are 85 per cent higher in organic soils. Researchers found higher vitamin C levels, higher mineral levels, more amino acids and less water in organic produce, which also contained lower levels of nitrates, nitrites and pesticide residues.

We are exposed to hundreds of different potential toxins in our food and environment. Many additives used in manufactured food and drink have been linked with health problems and are banned in organic food production.

Organic meat and poultry also offer health benefits. The routine use of antibiotics on animals to prevent illness is prohibited, and grass-fed animals have higher levels of CLA (a form of linoleic acid, an omega-6 fatty acid). Organic eggs also contain more essential fatty acids because the chickens eat a more natural diet.

The UK Food Standards Agency believes that there is not yet conclusive proof that organic food is better for us than inorganic produce. More research is needed, but some scientific studies already show the superiority of some types of organic food. For instance, a study at the University of Aberdeen showed that organic milk contained more omega-3 and vitamins than normal milk, and a ten-year study at the University of California proved that organic tomatoes were much higher in antioxidants than normal tomatoes.

Genetically modified (GM) foods are another controversial issue, and these, of course, are banned from organic farms. Although GM foods have not so far been proved to have any harmful effects, they have only been around for a few years, and some people are concerned that as yet unsuspected health problems may emerge at some time in the future.

If you would like to find out more about the health benefits of organic food, take a look at *Organic Farming, Food Quality and Human Health: A review of the evidence* by Shane Heaton (Soil Association, 2001).

There are, however, ways to ensure the food you eat is as nutritious as it can be – organic or not.

Organic produce is often difficult to get hold of and may be expensive. One alternative, if you live in the country, is a farm shop or farmers' market. Locally grown food should be fresher and therefore more nutritious than supermarket produce, which may have been transported thousands of miles to reach you. If you are a townie, use a local greengrocer and buy only produce that is in season.

When buying inorganic produce, always wash it well before use. Peel fruits such as apples and pears and always peel carrots, which frequently test positive for pesticide residues.

You may be able to find an organic box scheme, which will deliver fresh fruit and vegetables to your door once a week. This is particularly useful if you find shopping difficult. The Soil

Association can provide you with a list of box schemes, farm shops, farmers' markets and retailers (see Useful addresses).

If you have a friend or family member who is a keen gardener or who has an allotment, ask if he or she can supply you with fresh produce. Many gardeners nowadays use natural means of pest control; in any case, there will probably be less pesticide on home-grown fruit and vegetables than on supermarket purchases.

It is possible to grow some of your own food even if you are disabled or don't have a proper garden. You can grow all sorts of things in pots and planters, from salad leaves, herbs and tomatoes to strawberries and small fruit trees. All you need is a sunny patio, or even a table indoors in front of a south-facing window. Or why not turn the conservatory into a greenhouse? I've successfully grown peppers indoors on a wide sunny windowsill, and salad leaves and herbs in planters on the patio. Just remember that growing plants need regular watering, so if you can't manage this yourself, you may need some help.

Getting the balance right

Meals should be based round pasta, rice, potatoes, bread or cereal; then add a portion of fruit or vegetables and some protein – dairy products, meat, fish, chicken or pulses. Anyone with MS should always be sure to eat enough protein, as too little can worsen muscle weakness or fatigue – 115 g (4 oz) of protein per person per meal is about right.

Sometimes people with MS are overweight, perhaps because they cannot exercise properly or because depression leads them to 'comfort eat'. If you need to lose weight, the healthy eating diet should help, because you will be eating less of the sugary, fatty, refined foods that pile on the calories.

Vegetarians

According to the Vegetarian Society, research shows that, compared with an omnivorous (meat-eating) diet, a varied vegetarian diet contains less saturated fat and cholesterol and more folate, fibre, antioxidants and phytochemicals. It is also likely to contain more than the recommended five a day fruit and vegetables. The Oxford

Vegetarian Survey, which compared the health of 6,000 vegetarians with that of 5,000 meat eaters over 12 years, reported that vegetarians were 40 per cent less at risk from cancer, 30 per cent less at risk from heart disease and 20 per cent less likely to meet a premature death from other causes than the meat eaters. In countries such as India where vegetable protein forms the staple diet, MS is virtually unknown.

In a vegetarian diet, eating the right combination of foods to achieve an adequate protein intake can be quite a challenge. It is important not to take the easy option and just add cheese to every dish, as this will lead to a diet containing too much fat. Learn how to use nuts, beans and pulses to enhance your meals – the recipes in this book will show you the way. Because vegetarians eat a more limited range of foods, you need to ensure that as much as possible of what you eat is fresh, good quality, unrefined food full of vitamins and minerals.

If you rely on carers

Anyone who has to rely on agency carers for meals will be aware that they never have enough time to cook a meal from scratch using fresh ingredients. In any case, many professional carers have had virtually no training in cookery or nutrition. Some are reluctant to use a hob or grill because a microwave is the only form of cooking apparatus they are familiar with. I have even come across a few who do not know how to operate a can opener! In the circumstances, microwave meals from the supermarket may seem the only viable option for dinner.

Some years ago, after I broke my leg and was unable to access my kitchen easily, I needed to use agency carers to help me prepare meals. Luckily it wasn't long before I discovered the direct payments scheme, which enabled me to appoint my own carer, someone who could cook and was willing to follow my instructions to produce the sort of food I needed for my particular diet. I also paid a local lady to make a loaf of gluten-free bread, some gluten-free muffins and a batch of soup for me each week. During that period I proved that, by organizing the right help, it is possible to follow a special diet and eat extremely well even if you are unable to do any cooking yourself.

Explain to whoever helps you with shopping and cooking that you are trying to improve your health by changing what you eat.

All that is required is buying a different range of food at the super-market and changing the menu slightly. Most people are eager to help once they realize the changes needed are not complicated and will benefit your health.

First of all, make some changes to your shopping list. These could include buying:

- wholemeal bread instead of white bread, and wholegrain and reduced-sugar cereals
- ham and cooked chicken from delicatessens rather than the cheap processed variety
- polyunsaturated margarine instead of butter
- skimmed milk rather than full-fat milk, natural yogurt rather than ice-cream and low-fat or cottage cheese rather than hard cheese
- fruit juice and bottled water in place of fruit squash and cola drinks
- sugar-free jams and marmalades or honey
- items for your larder such as tinned fish (tuna, salmon and sardines), tinned fruit in fruit juice (not syrup), reduced-sugar baked beans and some good-quality tinned or chilled soups – those containing lentils and beans are particularly good as they are both filling and nutritious
- some salad ingredients, such as tomatoes, cucumber, celery and punnets of salad cress, large potatoes for baking in the micro-wave and individual packets of mixed vegetables designed to be cooked in a microwave
- a selection of fresh fruit, dried fruit, small packets of nuts and raisins or a tub of olives from the delicatessen, wholegrain crackers (such as Ryvita) to spread with hummus (also from the deli) and additive-free fruit smoothies for snacks
- the healthier, low-fat ranges of ready meals, opting for those made with chicken and fish rather than beef and lamb (it's surprising just how large the difference in fat content can be between these ranges and the standard ones).

Using these ingredients, your carers can prepare simple, healthy meals for you. Here are some suggestions.

- **Breakfast** Porridge made in the microwave, cereal with skimmed milk and sultanas or raisins instead of sugar or wholemeal toast with honey or sugar-free jam and a glass of fruit juice.

- **Lunch** A sandwich filled with ham or chicken and salad or tuna with low-fat mayonnaise or mashed sardine with sliced tomato. Scrambled eggs on toast or a potato baked in the microwave and served with cottage cheese or baked beans and a salad. A really simple salad that requires absolutely no expertise to prepare is a few slices of cucumber, a quartered tomato and half a punnet of salad cress. Try a large bowl of soup served with bread and a low-fat margarine. Have a piece of fruit for pudding.
- **Dinner** A ready meal served with a portion of cooked vegetables. Finish with a dessert of tinned fruit with low-fat custard or natural yogurt, a small bowl of muesli with milk or yogurt or another piece of fruit, such as half a small melon.

And finally . . .

A few words about all those things we love, but which can do us harm if we overindulge.

Caffeine

Caffeine, which is found in coffee, tea, cola, chocolate, energy drinks and some medicines, has a drug-like effect on the body. It is a diuretic, so it may make bladder problems worse. It is also a stimulant, causing the release of adrenaline into the body. This may prevent you relaxing properly, and too much could make your blood pressure rise. If consumed in large quantities, it can become addictive and can even cause heart attacks in otherwise healthy young people. In some people it can also cause mood swings, tremors, headaches, palpitations, insomnia and tingling in the arms and legs. Research in the USA has also found that caffeine makes it more difficult for the body to control acute inflammation.

If you consume a lot of caffeine on a daily basis, and especially if you suspect you may be addicted to it, you should consider cutting your intake. Reduce your consumption gradually to avoid withdrawal symptoms such as headaches. Start by replacing some cups of tea or coffee with the decaffeinated variety. After a week or so, you can substitute herbal teas for the decaffeinated drinks; there are some very exotic flavours available nowadays. Redbush makes an acceptable alternative to tea, and roasted chicory is a good coffee substitute. You could also try Barleycup if you are not avoiding gluten.

Of course, if you limit your coffee intake to, say, one cup a day and do not try to use it as a substitute for food when your energy is low, you may find you do not have a problem with caffeine.

Chocolate

Chocolate is a high-fat product, and all the paler varieties contain full-fat milk or cream and quite a lot of sugar. According to Jonathan Brostoff, Professor of Allergic and Environmental Health at King's College, London, there is limited evidence that some MS patients may be particularly susceptible to something in chocolate, and that this may play a part in developing their MS.

One Dutch medic, Dr Anna Maas, has had a great deal of success treating people with MS by removing from their diet chocolate and other substances such as cola and caffeine, which could cause an adverse reaction. She speculates that people with MS may lack an enzyme which is needed to metabolize chocolate properly.

On the other hand, recent research has shown that the flavonoids in dark chocolate helped reduce inflammation in heart attack and stroke victims. Since inflammation is a feature of MS, some people are now suggesting that eating small amounts of dark chocolate every day might well benefit people with MS. Dark chocolate contains more flavonoids than the paler dairy chocolate and also more than red wine, but has a much lower fat and sugar content.

If – like many people today – you're a bit of a chocoholic, this will come as good news to you. If, however, like me, you feel worse after eating chocolate, you may opt to try cutting it out altogether for a while and see if your health improves.

Alcohol

You may think that if you stick to the recommended maximum weekly intake – 14 units per week for both women and men – you are unlikely to do yourself any harm (1 unit of alcohol is 1 pint of beer or lager, 1 glass of wine, 1 measure of spirits or 1 bottle of alcopop). These units should be spread out through the week and people should have at least two alcohol-free days a week. Advice from the Department of Health states that pregnant women or women trying to conceive should not drink alcohol at all. If they do choose to drink, to minimize the risk to the baby they should not drink more than 1–2 units of alcohol once or twice a week and should not get drunk. These guidelines, however, are intended for the average healthy adult. If you have MS, there are even more good reasons for cutting down on alcohol.

Alcohol can worsen MS symptoms such as difficulties with walking, co-ordination, speech, balance and memory. Remember, also, that MS can decrease your tolerance to alcohol, so it may take only a small amount to cause deterioration in your symptoms. It is a depressant, so if you are feeling low and have a drink to make you feel better, it may have the opposite effect. Like tea and coffee, alcohol is a diuretic and may exacerbate bladder problems. It inhibits the conversion process of EFAs, which are very important for people with MS (see pages 49–50). It can also destroy the body's supply of vitamin C and zinc, and a heavy drinker may need to take as much as 500 mg vitamin C per day to replace that destroyed by alcohol.

Don't forget either that most alcoholic drinks contain sugar and yeast, and some contain gluten as well, so alcohol consumption needs to be restricted on the Best Bet diet and the Wahls diet. Professor Jelinek believes that moderate quantities of red wine are the safest bet because of their beneficial antioxidant content.

As with chocolate, my advice would be to try cutting alcohol out completely for a few weeks, to see if this has any effect on your symptoms, and after that to drink only in moderation (a maximum of 2 units at a time and no more than 4 units per week).

Smoking

Research into smoking and MS suggests that smoking more than doubles your chances of getting MS, even after you have given it up. It may also help transform relapsing–remitting MS into progressive MS. There is also proof that MS progresses faster in smokers than in non-smokers.

Research also shows that, far from helping you cope with stress, smoking actually raises stress levels, so it can often make MS symptoms worse. It can make you more prone to respiratory illnesses such as bronchitis and pneumonia, which can be harder to recover from if you already have a chronic illness. Smoking lowers your skin temperature, so it makes you feel worse if you suffer from frozen hands or feet in cold weather.

Cigarette smoke contains a cocktail of poisonous chemicals including carbon monoxide, which attaches itself to the oxygen-carrying part of your red blood cells so they can't carry as much oxygen around your body. If you already suffer from MS fatigue, this will leave you with even less energy. There is not much point in using diet to improve your health if you continue to bombard your body with toxic chemicals from cigarettes. A single cigarette can destroy 25 mg of vitamin C in your body. Cancer, emphysema and cardiovascular disease are all linked to smoking. Do you really want to increase your burden of illness?

Giving up smoking could also save you a considerable amount of money, which could instead go towards good-quality food and supplements. There is a lot of help available nowadays for anyone who wants to quit smoking. Nicotine replacement therapy comes in several different forms and is available on prescription. There are also drugs such as Zyban that help, although they can have side effects.

E-cigarettes are a fairly recent innovation for those who want to stop smoking. Recent research by Public Health England came to the conclusion that e-cigarettes are 95 per cent less harmful to health than normal cigarettes, though they do still contain nicotine, which is addictive. Evidence suggests that, when combined with a 'stop smoking' scheme such as NHS Smokefree, they help most smokers to quit smoking. (For details of the NHS scheme, see page 147.)

Supplements for the healthy eating diet

Anyone eating a healthy diet containing both animal and vegetable protein should be consuming a wide variety of vitamins and minerals. However, you may like to consider taking extra therapeutic doses of vitamins and minerals as outlined in 'Supplements that can help MS' (see page 13). In particular, if you smoke, or drink more than 4 units of alcohol per week, you should also consider taking a vitamin C supplement.

Vegetarians may need to take a vitamin B_{12} supplement as this vitamin is only found in sufficient quantities in animal-based foods. Anyone taking doses of individual B vitamins such as B_{12} should also take a B complex supplement as the two work together.

Vegetarians are also often short of iron. Although iron can be found in wholegrain bread, dark-green leafy vegetables and some dried fruit, we get most of our iron from animal protein, particularly red meat. Your GP can test your iron levels and prescribe a supplement if you need one.

4

The low-fat diet

Nutritional therapists believe that the right kinds of fats, eaten in the right amounts, keep you healthy, while a diet that contains too much of the wrong fats is one of the major causes of degenerative diseases such as MS.

A low-fat diet, therefore, does not involve cutting out fatty foods altogether. You do need to eat some fat, but it needs to be the right sort. The type of fat you should cut down on drastically is saturated fat, which is harmful if eaten in large quantities. Meanwhile, you should increase your intake of essential fatty acids, which are extremely beneficial to health.

How can a low-fat diet help MS?

In the Western world over the past 200 years, there has been a steady increase in the consumption of saturated fats, found in red meat, dairy products and processed foods. At the same time, the number of cases of MS has steadily increased. The first man to link these two facts was Professor Roy Swank who, as far back as 1948, advocated a low-fat diet for people with MS. Swank believed that some individuals were more sensitive to saturated fats than others, and that in susceptible individuals an excess of fat in the blood-stream could eventually cause a breakdown in the blood–brain barrier leading to demyelination and formation of plaques.

Professor Swank monitored a large group of people with MS over a period of more than 30 years. He found that 95 per cent of the patients in his study who started out with only minimal disability and who consistently ate no more than 20 g (4 tsp, or 0.7 oz) of saturated fat a day remained only mildly disabled. Members of the group who accidentally or intentionally increased their fat intake began to deteriorate again. On the other hand, people who managed to reduce their fat intake to 10–15 g (2–3 tsp) per day did even better than those on 20 g per day. Professor Swank also observed that the 'good' dieters (who ate a maximum of 20 g of fat per day) ate more polyunsaturated oils, while the 'poor' dieters (who ate more than 20 g of fat per day) ate less of these oils.

'Good' dieters reported a decrease in fatigue over time and were also better able to cope with stress without deterioration. Those who were more disabled at the start of the study reported an increased sense of well-being and either stabilization of their condition or a slowing down of deterioration. This is the largest and longest study carried out so far on the effects of diet on MS.

Another researcher who has been crucial in expanding our knowledge of good and bad fats is the German scientist Johanna Budwig, who developed techniques for separating and identifying different types of fat in a drop of blood. She then compared blood samples from sick and healthy people and investigated their fat content. She observed that healthy people's blood always contained EFAs, while sick people lacked lipoproteins (a mixture of the EFA linoleic acid and proteins). She tried feeding an oil-protein diet to patients with chronic illnesses and some recovered completely. This led to her promoting flaxseed oil in nutritional therapy for many different chronic conditions, because it contains a good balance of omega-3 and omega-6 EFAs.

In the 1970s and 1980s more trials were carried out on diet and MS, this time with the emphasis on EFAs. In 1973, the *British Medical Journal* published the results of a study in which sunflower oil (a source of omega-6 EFAs) was given to people with the relapsing–remitting type of MS. Results suggested that the frequency, severity and duration of attacks were reduced in the group who took the sunflower oil.

In 1978 another trial, led by Dr David Bates, took place at Newcastle University. This trial involved 116 people with MS, divided into four groups. Group A were given evening primrose oil capsules; Group B took olive oil capsules; Group C were given sunflower margarine; and Group D got a placebo. After two years, the only difference in outcome in the four groups was that those taking the sunflower margarine reported shorter and less severe MS attacks. The evening primrose oil did not perform as well as expected in this trial. One reason could be that the subjects were not told to cut down on saturated fat, and it is now known that saturated fats can prevent proper metabolism of EFAs.

One trial that set out to correct this problem was that carried out at the Central Middlesex Hospital in the 1980s. The trial lasted three years and involved 83 people with MS. They were told to eat less saturated fat and more omega-3 and omega-6 EFAs. They were also given advice on vitamin and mineral supplementation and fibre intake. This 'optimum nutrition diet' produced a clear distinction in outcome between those who stuck faithfully to the diet, who did not get significantly worse, and those who lapsed from the diet, who did.

Professor Bates then investigated fish oil (an omega-3 EFA) as a treatment for MS. The results were less clear-cut, but still suggested people might benefit from eating food that contained both omega-3 and omega-6 oils.

Analysis of the results of the most significant trials involving EFAs and MS suggests that the lower the level of disability at the start of the trial, the higher the chance the person can prevent deterioration by taking polyunsaturated fats. If this is true, then those who alter their diet as soon as possible after diagnosis have the best chance of stabilizing their condition, though this should not put you off trying a diet if your diagnosis is some way behind you.

The MS diet trials to date are considered by many doctors to be too few and too small to prove the case. Undoubtedly, more work needs to be done, particularly since most of the subjects so far have had relapsing–remitting MS rather than the progressive form of the disease. However, the existing studies do – at the very least – suggest that a low-fat diet could be a promising self-help option for people with MS, and certainly this is backed up by anecdotal evidence.

The science behind the diet

Why are EFAs especially important for people with MS? EFAs are the main components of the membranes that surround all cells. They form part of the nucleus of each cell, which is the area containing the genetic 'master plan' for our bodies. EFAs are involved in oxidation, the 'burning' of food to produce energy, and govern our growth, mental state and sex hormones.

People with MS have been shown to have abnormalities in their red and white blood cells, but these can be corrected within one year if EFA supplements are taken.

EFAs form roughly 60 per cent of the brain; they are the building blocks of the central nervous system and essential for brain function. EFAs are also necessary for the manufacture of prostaglandins, hormone-like substances that help promote healing, dampen down an over-active immune system and enhance immune efficiency, thus improving resistance to infection.

There are several different families of unsaturated fatty acids. The most important are omega-3 and omega-6. Both are essential to human health but cannot be manufactured in the body. This is why they are called essential fatty acids (EFAs).

The omega-3 family – super-unsaturated fatty acids

- **Alpha-linolenic acid (ALA or LNA)** – the richest source of LNA is flax seeds (also known as linseeds). Half the EFA in flax seeds is LNA. It is also found in soya beans, walnuts and dark-green leaves.
- **Stearidonic acid (SDA)** is found in blackcurrant seeds.
- **Eicosapentaenoic acid (EPA) and docosahexaenoic acid (DHA)** are found in oily fish such as salmon, trout, mackerel and sardines, which contain up to 30 per cent EFAs.

The omega-6 family – polyunsaturated fatty acids

- **Linoleic acid (LA)** is found in safflower oil, sunflower oil, soya beans, walnuts, pumpkins and sesame and flax seeds.
- **Gamma-linolenic acid (GLA)** is found in borage oil (also known as starflower oil), blackcurrant seed oil and evening primrose oil.
- **Dihomo-y-linolenic acid (DGLA)** is found in breastmilk.
- **Arachidonic acid (AA)** is found in meat.

The omega-9 family – monounsaturated fatty acids

- **Oleic acid (OA)** is found in olive oil, almonds, avocados, peanuts, pecans, cashew nuts and macadamia nuts. Oleic acid has a neutral effect on us. It is not an essential fatty acid because – unlike the omega-3 and omega-6 fatty acids – it can be produced by the body.

The EFA pathway

Omega-3 and omega-6 fatty acids are metabolized in the body into more complicated unsaturated fatty acids, which are the ones needed by the brain. This is called the EFA pathway. Things that can interfere with the EFA pathway include:

- too much saturated or hydrogenated fat
- too much sugar
- too much alcohol
- a lack of vitamins and minerals (especially B_6, zinc and magnesium)
- exposure to pollution
- smoking.

It has been suggested that people with MS may have difficulty converting the original fatty acids into their more complex forms. One solution could be eating more of those foods that already contain the more complex fatty acids, such as evening primrose oil, oats, liver, kidneys, fish and seafood.

Why saturated fats are a problem

As well as interfering with the EFA pathway, saturated fats can cause other problems. For instance, they have a tendency to stick together to form sticky platelets that can turn into blood clots and lead to strokes or heart disease. Because the blood is stickier, it doesn't flow as well through our veins and arteries and this in turn decreases the supply of oxygen to our tissues.

However, it's not just the saturated fats we eat directly in the form of meat or dairy products that we need to worry about. The sugar we consume also turns to saturated fat in our bodies, and starchy foods turn into glucose (another form of sugar) as they are digested. Refined starches such as white flour or white rice are more likely to end up as saturated fats than whole grains such as wholemeal flour or brown rice.

Processed fats

Hydrogenation was invented in the 1930s, paving the way for the first margarines. Unsaturated fats and oils are reacted with hydrogen at high temperatures to create a product that is convenient to use and has a very long shelf life. Unfortunately, as well as removing almost all the nutrients from the product, hydrogenation can also produce toxic substances such as trans-fatty acids. Like saturated fats, trans-fatty acids make blood more sticky. They also inhibit EFAs from doing their job effectively. Most UK supermarkets have now removed hydrogenated oils from their own brands, and current UK regulations require that hydrogenated and trans-fats should be declared in the ingredients list of all products.

The following diet is based on that pioneered by Professor Roy Swank.

The diet

Cut down on saturated fat

Eat a maximum of 15 g (3 tsp) saturated fat per day. These fats are hard at room temperature and are found in:

- red meat (beef, lamb and pork, for example; a maximum of 85 g (3 oz) per week is allowed, after the first year);
- animal fats such as lard, dripping and suet;
- processed meats such as sausages, bacon and salami;
- full-fat dairy products such as full-cream milk, hard cheese and butter (skimmed milk, low-fat cheeses, such as cottage cheese and quark, and low-fat yogurt are permitted);
- fatty poultry such as duck and geese;
- some nuts (Brazil nuts, peanuts, macadamia nuts and coconuts);
- some vegetable fats (coconut oil and palm oil);
- manufactured foods such as crisps, cakes, chocolate, pies, biscuits;
- eggs – buy organic free-range rather than battery-farmed eggs if you can, as they contain beneficial EFAs, and eat a maximum of three eggs per week, no more than one egg in any one day (egg whites are virtually fat-free so are unrestricted).

Cut out processed fats and oils

This means eliminating any food that contains hydrogenated fats or trans fats and refined cooking oils. Margarines are the main culprits for hydrogenated fats, but the label won't always tell you this. It's easier to search out the products that state clearly, 'Does not contain hydrogenated fats'. Examples are Bertolli margarine (made from olive oil) and Pure Vegetable Spread (made from sunflower oil). Alternatively, you could do as the Italians do and spread olive oil instead of margarine on bread.

When choosing oils for cooking or using in salad dressings, buy the ones that are labelled 'cold-pressed' or 'unrefined' oils. These oils will not have been subjected to the same high temperatures and chemical processes as off-the-shelf cooking oils, and retain their original health benefits. Olive oil has a different labelling system from the other oils: the pure unrefined variety is called 'extra virgin' and you can buy it in supermarkets, but other unrefined oils such as sunflower or sesame seed are usually only stocked in health food shops.

Don't use unrefined oils to cook food at very high temperatures, as this destroys their nutrients and creates toxic substances. Stir-frying over a high heat is acceptable, because it's a very quick process. Otherwise – when cooking onions, for instance – 'sweat' foods in oil in a covered pan over a very low heat for up to 10 minutes. Never deep-fry food. This process changes the molecules from the unsaturated type into the saturated trans-fatty acids that are so bad for your health.

Table 4.1 shows the fat content of some common foods.

Eat more EFAs

On the low-fat diet, you need to make sure you get enough omega-6 and omega-3 EFAs. However, while there is general agreement that it is important to take the right ratio of omega-6 to omega-3, there seems to be some dispute among professionals as to what exactly

Table 4.1 Fat content of common foods

Each of these quantities of food is equivalent to 1 tsp (5g) unsaturated fat.

- 90 g (3 oz) tuna in oil, drained
- 60 g (2 oz) trout
- 60 g (2 oz) salmon
- 30 g (1 oz) sardines in oil, drained
- 30 g (1 oz) herring or mackerel
- 2 tsp unhydrogenated peanut butter
- 2 tsp tahini spread
- 45 g (1½ oz) avocado
- 3 medium black olives
- 6 medium green olives

Oils (i.e. sunflower, olive or flaxseed oil) are pure unsaturated fat, so 1 tsp oil = 1 tsp unsaturated fat.

is the right ratio. Three parts omega-6 to one part omega-3 is the ratio normally recommended for a low-fat diet. Dr Ashton Embry, promoter of the Best Bet diet, advocates a ratio nearer 2:1. Udo Erasmus, author of *Fats that Heal, Fats that Kill*, uses a 1:1 ratio in his oils, the balance found in flaxseed oil, which Johanna Budwig believed to be so beneficial to health. The most recent research into EFAs and MS, carried out in Cyprus in 2013, also suggested a ratio of 1:1 omega-3 to omega-6. If you are unsure which ratio to go for, why not ask the advice of a nutritional therapist?

It is difficult to achieve the right balance of EFAs by diet alone, so supplementation with EFA capsules is recommended (see 'Supplements for the low-fat diet', page 56). In addition, include all the following foods in your diet – these are the low-fat superfoods that will boost your EFA intake naturally:

- linseeds, pumpkin seeds, sunflower seeds, sesame seeds
- walnuts, almonds, pine nuts
- avocados and dark-green leafy vegetables
- oily fish such as herring, tuna, salmon, mackerel and sardines
- unrefined oils such as sunflower oil and flaxseed oil.

Try also to eat regularly those foods that contain the more complex fatty acids: oats, liver, kidneys, white fish, seafood.

You need to monitor your intake of unsaturated fats as well as saturated ones. The allowance of unsaturated fats is 20–50 g (4–10 tsp) per day. See Table 4.1 (page 52) for the fat content of some common foods. Try and spread your fat allowance throughout the day, and if you eat a high-fat food at one meal, balance it with a low-fat dish at the next meal. Any oil used in cooking should be measured out carefully; alternatively, use an oil spray and a non-stick pan. Remember – moderation is the keyword, even with beneficial fats.

Foods containing EFAs need to be stored carefully. Unrefined oils such as sunflower oil or extra virgin olive oil should be kept in a cool dark place, such as a cupboard or larder. Flaxseed oil, which is particularly vulnerable to light and air, should be kept in an opaque sealed container in the fridge and used within three weeks.

Keep nuts in a sealed plastic container in the freezer for up to a month to stop them going rancid. Seeds also need to be kept in sealed containers in a cupboard and eaten within a month.

Replace refined starchy foods with whole grains

There are several reasons for this. Both sugars and refined starchy foods turn into saturated fats in our bodies (see 'Why saturated fats are a problem' on page 50), whereas wholegrain foods are absorbed more slowly and are less likely to turn into fats. Whole grains also contain nutrients that are used in the EFA conversion process and fibre, which helps our digestive system function properly.

Identify food intolerances

If you have a sensitivity to dairy products, eating the low-fat varieties won't make you feel better. Likewise, if you are wheat intolerant, eating wholemeal bread may actually make you feel worse than eating refined white bread. It is wise, therefore, to identify any food intolerances before you start your diet (see 'Finding out if you have food intolerances', pages 21–2).

The vegan option

A vegan diet (no meat, poultry, fish or dairy products) is the vegetarian version of the low-fat diet. Many of the foods vegans eat every day – such as nuts, seeds, whole grains – contain the EFAs that are a crucial part of a low-fat diet. Remember, though, that if you are underweight or regularly undertake strenuous exercise, a vegan diet may not provide you with a sufficiently wide range of protein foods.

You should eat as wide a range of vegan protein foods as possible. These include nuts, seeds and nut milk; pulses (peas, beans, lentils); mushrooms; tofu; Quorn; and quinoa.

You can also eat:

- all fruit and vegetables – as wide a range as possible
- whole grains – rice, millet, buckwheat, bulgur wheat, couscous
- bread and pasta made from unrefined flours
- unrefined oils
- dairy-free margarines and vegan cheese made from sunflower and soya
- soya, rice and oat milk, soya yogurts, soya ice-cream
- non-dairy chocolate or carob.

Vegan superfoods

When you have cut out a whole food group such as animal protein, you need to ensure that the foods you do eat are as packed with nutrients as possible. These vegan superfoods should be eaten two or three times a week for maximum benefits.

- **Mushrooms** These help decrease inflammation in the body. They contain sulphur, antioxidants, vitamin D, B vitamins and other nutrients. Sulphur helps create neurotransmitters and removes toxins from the body. Gilenya, the first oral drug for relapsing–remitting MS, is derived from a type of mushroom.
- **Sea vegetables (seaweed)** These contain more minerals than any other food source. Some contain up to ten times as much calcium as milk and eight times as much iron as beef. Sea vegetables come in several different varieties and are available in health food shops and some supermarkets. An easy way to eat them is to add them to soups and stews.
- **Sprouted seeds** These are young green plants germinated from seeds. They contain high concentrations of antioxidant vitamins and minerals, which help fight free radicals. They are also full of protein, enzymes, fibre and nucleic acids, which are anti-ageing factors. The salad cress you can buy in punnets are sprouted seeds and so are the beansprouts used in Chinese cooking. Eat them raw in salads or add them to stir-fries just before serving, as cooking destroys their vital nutrients.
- **Quinoa** Pronounced 'keenwa', this is a South American grain that contains all nine essential amino acids normally only found in animal products, as well as many minerals. It is a complete low-fat protein and is easier to digest than meat.
- **Seeds and berries** Three plant foods that have only recently become readily available are goji berries, acai berries and chia seeds. Both types of berries contain omega-3 fatty acids (otherwise found mainly in fish). Goji berries, like quinoa, are a complete source of protein and contain all the amino acids. Chia seeds also contain fibre, protein and minerals. For tasty ideas on how to incorporate these superfoods into your diet, I recommend *Deliciously Ella* by Ella Woodward, who overcame a chronic illness by changing to a vegan diet.

Supplements for the low-fat diet

EFAs

You should be taking both GLA (omega-6), in the form of evening primrose oil (EPO) or starflower oil, and fish oil (omega-3) The recommended dose varies, but you could start with 4–6 g (1 tsp) EPO (or 2–3 g starflower oil) and 1–2 g fish oil per day. Choose fish oils made from high-fat cold-water fish such as salmon. This is better than cod liver oil, which is high in vitamin A, may contain toxic substances and is subject to pollution. Vegans can substitute flaxseed oil for evening primrose oil and fish oil, as it contains both omega-3 and omega-6.

Additional vitamins and minerals are required to help metabolize EFAs into prostaglandins:

- zinc
- magnesium
- calcium
- biotin, vitamin B_3 and B_6
- vitamin C

- 15 mg per day
- 600 mg per day
- 1,200 mg per day
- 1 x vitamin B complex per day
- 1,000 mg per day

Vegans should also take 1,000 iu of vitamin B_{12} per day and additional iron.

5

The Best Bet diet

The Best Bet diet was pioneered by a Canadian scientist, Dr Ashton Embry, whose son has MS. He believes some of the protein foods that form part of the modern Western diet can trigger an immunological response in those people with a genetic susceptibility to MS and lack of sufficient vitamin D also contributes to the problem.

Dr Embry started by looking at the geographical spread of the disease. Research shows that the incidence of MS is dependent on distance from the equator. The populations with the highest proportion of MS cases are those furthest away from the equator, and this applies even within the same country (for instance, there are more people with MS in the north of Scotland than in the south of England). This seems to suggest that MS might be linked with lack of sunshine, which is our main source of vitamin D_3. Although there are areas that have low sunshine levels and a low rate of MS, these tend to be areas where the population eat a lot of oily fish – the other main source of vitamin D. Dr Embry began to wonder if vitamin D might play a part in protecting people against MS.

He also believes that MS has been triggered by the agricultural and industrial changes of the recent past. Some 5,000 years ago, our ancestors spent most of their lives in the open air and ate a diet of freshly caught meat, fish and wildfowl, together with nuts, seeds, fruits and edible plants. This is known as the Paleo diet. Since then, we have kept farmed animals and poultry and cultivated grains such as wheat and barley. All this has happened in a relatively short space of time in evolutionary terms, and it is possible that some people cannot cope very well with these more 'modern' foods. More recently still, we have moved from living mainly in the countryside to living mainly in towns and cities and have begun to eat large quantities of manufactured processed foods.

These environmental changes suggest that the main factors affecting MS could be:

- the introduction of new proteins into our diets, such as cow's milk, gluten grains and legumes;
- deficiencies in vitamin D, caused by spending less time outside in the open air than in the past;
- a deficiency in omega-3 fatty acids and antioxidants, due to not eating enough fish and plant foods.

According to the theory behind the Best Bet diet, the MS process starts when particles of undigested food escape through the gut walls and into the bloodstream (known as 'leaky gut syndrome'). The immune system sees the food particles as invaders and starts attacking them. However, the protein molecules in certain foods are similar to the myelin that sheathes the nerves. This is called molecular mimicry and it causes the immune system to attack the myelin as well as the food particles.

Various proteins from cow's milk, gluten and legumes have been shown to be molecular mimics of the protein in myelin. Gluten is already known to be at the root of two autoimmune diseases, coeliac disease and *Dermatitis herpetiformis*, and the highest incidence of MS occurs in areas where a lot of gluten is consumed. There is a similar correlation between MS and milk consumption.

There are three main components of the diet:

- avoiding foods such as dairy products, gluten grains and legumes that are molecularly similar to myelin and activate the immune reaction;
- taking a range of supplements to help dampen down the auto-immune reaction, aid healing of the 'leaky gut' and ensure adequate nutrients;
- detecting any additional food sensitivities, so that these foods can be either rotated or avoided altogether (foods you are sensitive to can make a leaky gut worse and increase immune reactions).

The science behind the Best Bet diet

Ashton Embry believes MS may be a deficiency disease caused by lack of vitamin D, and suggests it could be eliminated by supplementing children with vitamin D in the same way rickets (another deficiency disease) was banished in the last century by giving children cod liver oil. Recent research seems to support this theory.

There has also been some research into the sensitivity of people with MS to proteins such as cow's milk and gluten. Scientists have observed that mice – who have a similar immune system to ours – get an MS-type illness if injected with milk proteins. Now researchers in Canada have found that the protein in cow's milk is an important risk factor in the development of both MS and another autoimmune disease, type 1 diabetes. Both diseases share genetic similarities and similar patterns of geographical distribution. Both have a long period of 'silent illness' before initial symptoms appear. If this research can be duplicated on a larger scale, it could suggest that for people who are particularly at risk, a milk-free diet might prevent later development of both diseases.

Trials of the Best Bet diet

A scientific trial of the Best Bet diet, funded by Ashton Embry's charity DIRECT-MS, took place at Ninewells Hospital in Dundee in 2007–8. This pilot study was a randomized controlled single-blind test to compare the Best Bet diet to the healthy eating diet in patients with relapsing–remitting MS. The object was to see whether the Best Bet diet (a) delayed progression and (b) controlled symptoms. There were 22 participants, 11 on the Best Bet diet and 11 on the healthy eating diet, and the trial lasted for a year. The results showed that after 12 months, those on the Best Bet diet had a lower rate of brain shrinkage, less change in disability and significantly better scores on MS function and vision tests. It is difficult to draw conclusions from such a small study, but it does suggest that it would be well worth carrying out a larger trial in the future to confirm these results.

The diet

Foods you should avoid completely

You should avoid any foods that contain gluten, the protein found in wheat, rye and barley. This means avoiding most shop-bought bread, cakes, biscuits, pies, pizza and so on, which all contain wheat flour, plus many other products that contain hidden cereals (see Table 5.1 for a list of foods that you should suspect contain wheat or gluten). For the purposes of this diet, refined and unrefined gluten grains are equally bad for you so read food labels carefully

Table 5.1 Foods and products that may contain wheat or gluten

Baked beans
Baking powder
Beer
Biscuits
Burgers
Cakes and muffins
Chocolate bars
Chutney and pickles
Communion wafers
Cornflakes
Curry powder
Dry roasted nuts
Food cooked in breadcrumbs
Instant oat breakfast cereals
Malt vinegar
Margarine (may contain wheatgerm oil)
Medicines (wheatflour is used as a binder)
Mustard
Noodles
Pasta sauces and sauce mixes
Pâtés
Processed meat
Ready-made soups
Salad dressings and mayonnaise
Sausages
Soya sauce
Spice mixes
Stock cubes and gravy powder
Sweets
Vitamin tablets
White pepper

Table 5.2 Ingredients listed on food labels that may contain wheat and gluten

Bran
Cereal
Corn or cornflour, cornstarch
Couscous
Durum flour
Edible starch
Filler
Flour (type unspecified)
Food starch
Malt
Modified starch
MSG (often made from wheatstarch)
Rusk
Textured vegetable protein (TVP)
Semolina
Spelt flour (an ancient type of wheat)
Thickener
Triticale (a wheat–rye hybrid)

Table 5.3 Terms used on food labels that indicate contents may include milk and foods that often contain milk

Terms for ingredients that indicate contents may include milk

Cassein/casseinate
Curds
Ghee
Lactic acid
Lactose
Whey

Foods that often contain milk

Acidopholus
Biscuits
Cakes and muffins
Chocolate bars
Chorizo
Custard powder
Gluten-free bread, cakes and biscuits
Margarines
Mayonnaise
Medicines and food supplements
Muesli
Pasta sauces and sauce mixes
Pastry
Pâtés
Ready-made soups
Sweet and savoury pies and pastries
Sweets, particularly caramel and fudge

Table 5.4 Plants classified as legumes

Legumes are the fruits or seeds of anything that comes in a pod.

- All types of beans, including cocoa beans and coffee beans
- All types of lentils
- All types of peas, including chickpeas
- Gram flour, which is derived from chickpeas and is used to make poppadoms
- Alfalfa (often sold as sprouting seeds)
- Carob
- Chocolate (made from cocoa beans)
- Guar gum (a stabilizer used in gluten-free baking)
- Liquorice
- Peanuts
- Tamarind (used in Asian cooking)
- Vanilla (small amounts may be used in recipes, but don't use every day)

(see Table 5.2). Oats, which contain proteins similar to gluten, may be a problem for some people, so go cautiously with them.

Also avoid all dairy products, including cow's milk, sheep's milk and goat's milk, and all products made from them, such as cheese, yogurt, butter, ice-cream and dairy chocolate, even the low-fat varieties, plus all products that contain hidden dairy products (see Table 5.3 for terms for milk products that can be found as ingredients on food labels and a list of foods that often contain milk).

Avoid all legumes, including peas, beans, lentils and peanuts, and all products made from legumes, such as soya milk, soya sauce, tofu, bean curd (see Table 5.4 for a full list of legumes).

Obviously, also avoid any food to which you are sensitive. (See pages 21–2 for details of how to identify food intolerances.)

Foods that are restricted

Fats

There are two types of fat: saturated and unsaturated. Saturated fats are the ones you need to cut down on drastically. In the Best Bet diet, you are allowed a maximum of 80 g (16 tsp) of fat per day, of which no more than 18 g (3 tsp) should be saturated fat. Saturated fats are found in red meat such as lamb, beef and pork; animal fats such as lard, dripping and suet; processed meat such as sausages and salami; dairy products; some poultry, such as duck and geese; some nuts; and some vegetable fats, such as coconut milk and palm oil. In addition, any fat labelled as 'hydrogenated' is saturated.

Unsaturated fats are the omega fats. (For a fuller explanation of omega fats, see page 49.) You should aim to eat more omega-3 fats (found in oily fish) and omega-9 fats (found in olive oil) and less of the omega-6 polyunsaturated fats (found in margarines and seeds). A daily intake of unsaturated fat of 20–65 g (4–13 tsp) is allowed. To achieve a proper balance of the fat types, the suggested amounts per day of the four types are:

- 40 g (8 tsp) monounsaturated fat
- 18 g (2½ tsp) saturated fat
- 14 g (2 tsp) omega-6
- 8 g (1 tsp) omega-3.

As with the low-fat diet, because of the difficulty of achieving this ratio with diet alone, supplementation with fish oil and flaxseed oil is recommended (see 'Supplements for the Best Bet diet', pages 65–6). However, note that this ratio of fats is different from that suggested for the low-fat diet.

Meat

To help limit fat consumption, only one portion of red meat (beef, lamb, pork, liver or kidneys) is allowed per week. This should be either grilled or roasted using a rack, so that any excess fat can be poured away. Ham and bacon, both processed meats, should also be restricted.

Eggs

Eggs have a high fat content and are highly allergenic, so should be eaten no more than twice a week. Avoid products that contain egg, and replace battery eggs with organic free-range eggs for their increased EFA content.

Yeast

Yeast is another highly allergenic food. Although there are small quantities of yeast in such products as stock cubes and tinned soups, most of the yeast in your diet is likely to come from bread.

You can restrict your yeast intake by making gluten-free (GF) soda breads (see page 132), which are much easier and quicker to make than yeasted breads. You should also avoid yeasted spreads such as Marmite or Vegemite.

Non-gluten grains

It is recommended that you eat only moderate quantities of non-gluten grains such as rice, as these grains also contain relatively 'new' proteins, which may disagree with some people. They can also increase gut permeability.

Sugars

Avoid sugar where possible. Eat honey or maple syrup instead.

Alcohol

Beer contains gluten and wine has a high sugar and yeast content, while spirits are distilled from grains. On the plus side, red wine does contain valuable antioxidants, so red wine (in moderation) is probably your best option.

Foods you can eat freely

- **Fish** All types of freshwater and deep sea fish.
- **Seafood** Prawns, cockles, mussels, lobster, crab, squid (unless you know you have a problem with shellfish or your cholesterol level is high).
- **Poultry** Chicken and turkey breast, but not the skin. The other parts of these birds also have a higher fat content, but may be eaten occasionally.
- **Game** Examples are rabbit and venison (but avoid frozen rabbit from other countries as it may be of poor quality).
- **Dairy-free spreads** For example, Pure Sunflower Spread. (Check they are also soya- and wheat-free and contain no hydrogenated or trans fats.)
- **Milk** Rice milk and nut milk.
- **Gluten-free foods** Bread and bread mixes, cakes, biscuits and crackers, so long as they contain no soya, dairy products, eggs, sugar or yeast.
- **Nuts** Walnuts, almonds, pine nuts, chestnuts, hazelnuts, cashews

and pistachios; also spreads made out of these nuts, such as almond butter. Avoid the high-fat nuts, such as Brazil and macadamia, and peanuts, which are a type of legume.

- **Seeds** Pumpkin, sesame, sunflower, flax seeds (linseeds) and chia seeds.
- **Vegetable protein foods** Quorn products that are milk- and gluten-free, but not textured vegetable protein, which contains soya and may also contain gluten.
- **Oils** Olive, sunflower, flaxseed, walnut and sesame oils.
- **Gluten-free whole grains** Rice, wild rice, millet, buckwheat, quinoa, polenta.
- **Fruit** All kinds.
- **Vegetables and herbs** All kinds.
- **Flours** Rice, millet, buckwheat, potato, tapioca and maize flours, arrowroot and amaranth and gluten-free cornflour.
- **Seasonings** The following may be used if gluten-free: all types of vinegar except malt vinegar, Worcestershire sauce, tomato purée, garlic purée or garlic in oil, mustard, curry powder, ground spices, salt and black pepper (not white pepper).

Supplements for the Best Bet diet

The following supplements are designed to work in conjunction with the Best Bet diet. This is an abridged list to give you an idea of the range of suggested supplements (you can find the full list at <www.direct-ms.org.). It would be wise to discuss the regime with a qualified nutritional therapist or healthcare professional before you start in order to check that none of the supplements will interact with any medication you are taking.

Essential supplements

- 6,000–8,000 iu vitmin D_3 (for more information on how to work out how much vitamin D you need, and how to take it, see page 15).
- 5 g omega-3 fatty acids EPA and DHA from salmon oil capsules
- 1 tbsp flaxseed oil
- 1,000–1,200 mg calcium
- 500–600 mg magnesium

Other basic supplements

- 5,000 iu vitamin A (note that this is the maximum safe daily dose from all sources)
- 100 mg vitamin B complex
- 1–2 mg vitamin B$_{12}$
- 1 g vitamin C
- 400 iu vitamin E
- 25–50 mg zinc
- 200 mcg selenium
- 200 mcg iodine
- 120 mg *Ginkgo biloba*
- 60–90 mg co-enzyme Q10
- 1,200 mg alpha-lipoic acid
- 2–3 acidopholus capsules with each meal (different makes vary in strength – see guidance on page 18)

Choosing gluten-free and dairy-free products

Finding food products that are free from gluten, wheat, dairy, egg, yeast and soya can be quite challenging. It is getting easier, though, partly through new EU laws on food labelling and partly through manufacturers' growing awareness of food sensitivities.

Coeliac UK, the charity that represents those who cannot eat gluten, publishes an invaluable directory of gluten-free products, updated yearly. Be aware, though, that you will still have to check the labels on gluten-free products to see if they contain other foods you wish to avoid. There are now many companies manufacturing gluten-free foods. Some are available in supermarkets and health shops and some can be ordered direct from specialist internet retailers (see Useful addresses).

Confusingly, not all gluten-free products are also wheat-free. Some are made from a form of wheat flour that has had the gluten removed. Look for the products that are clearly labelled 'wheat-free' and 'gluten-free' (see Table 5.1, page 60). Tables 5.2 and 5.3 (page 61) show lists of ingredients you should look out for when buying food items because they indicate that either gluten or dairy may be present.

Bread

Most gluten-free breads use yeast as a raising agent, but there are a few that use an alternative raising agent. The best of these, I have found, is Orgran bread mix, which can be made successfully in both a conventional oven and a breadmaker. Orgran is an Australian company that makes a whole range of organic gluten-free foods such as bread, pasta, flour, pastry and pizza mixes, porridge and muesli. For details of UK suppliers, see page 148.

Margarines

Most margarines contain whey powder from milk, or wheatgerm oil, but Pure Sunflower Spread (available from health food shops and larger supermarkets) is milk-free and has the added bonus of being made from unhydrogenated oils.

Other products

Marigold Vegetable Bouillon Powder is a stock powder that contains no yeast. An alternative is Kallo Organic Vegetable Stock Cubes.

Xanthan gum, Orgran No Gluten, and GF baking powder are all useful in gluten-free baking, and Doves Farm make a good range of gluten-free flours.

6

The Overcoming MS diet

Professor George Jelinek first started looking into treatment options for multiple sclerosis when he himself was diagnosed with the disease in 1999.

As a professor of emergency medicine and the editor of a medical journal, he was only interested in treatments that were backed up by scientific evidence. As he worked his way through a huge number of scientific papers, he began to feel the evidence suggested that lifestyle changes were more effective than drugs in treating chronic Western diseases such as MS. As he points out in his book *Overcoming Multiple Sclerosis: An evidence-based guide to recovery*, such changes empower people with the condition and improve their quality of life while avoiding the side effects of medication, as well as helping to avoid other serious medical conditions.

Professor Jelinek finally came to the conclusion that dietary fat intake markedly affects the function of the immune system. He found that saturated (animal) fats and omega-6 fatty acids excite the immune system, while omega-3 fatty acids, found in fish and flax seeds, dampen it down. Omega-9 fatty acids (olive oil) appear to be neutral. Unsaturated fatty acids (omega-3, omega-6 and omega-9) all help to prevent degeneration.

He then looked at studies of disease distribution and concluded that the evidence suggested MS is more prevalent in countries where more animal fat is eaten and less evident where more fish is eaten. His research also pointed to a strong link between cow's milk consumption and MS, and suggested that fish-based and vegetarian diets played a protective role in MS. Unlike Ashton Embry and Terry Wahls, however, he remained unconvinced that there was any association between either gluten or legumes and MS.

Having looked at clinical studies that investigated the relationship of diet to MS and discovered Professor Roy Swank's 34-year study of MS patients who cut their fat intake, he then began to study the role of vitamin D in MS. He found epidemiological, laboratory, animal and human research that pointed to vitamin D deficiency as a cause of MS. He also noted that a seasonal variation in the activity of the disease seemed to be linked to the seasonal variation in sunlight levels.

Based on this research, Professor Jelinek developed a recovery programme involving a plant-based wholefood diet with added fish and seafood, supplements such as omega-3 and B complex vitamins, and an adequate intake of vitamin D from either sunlight or supplementation. He also recommends daily meditation, regular exercise and counselling to resolve any deep-rooted emotional issues.

He himself has been following this programme successfully since shortly after his diagnosis. Since 2000 he has had no relapses and no deterioration. In 2002 he began to run retreats for people with MS in Australia and New Zealand (and more recently in the UK), in which participants get the opportunity to sample the dietary regime and lifestyle changes that he recommends. His website, <http://overcomingms.org>, now has an active community of several thousand members. For his work with MS and emergency medicine, Professor Jelinek has twice been a finalist in the Australian of the Year awards.

Controversially, he suggests that it is possible not just to slow down or halt the progress of the disease, but to make a full recovery. He sees recovery as a healing process rather than a cure, because the person with MS is healing him- or herself through lifestyle changes rather than relying on a treatment or medical procedure provided by a third party. His latest book, *Recovering from Multiple Sclerosis*, published in 2013, tells the real-life stories of people of different ages and backgrounds from around the world who, after modifying their diets and changing other aspects of their lives, have regained their health.

The diet

Foods to avoid

- All saturated fats.
- Refined and manufactured fats (such as trans fats and hydrogenated fats), as well as coconut oil, which is a saturated fat.
- All forms of meat and poultry.

- Eggs (egg whites are acceptable).
- All dairy products (milk, butter, cheese, yogurt and so on) from any animal. (See Table 5.3 on page 61 for details of foods that may contain milk.) Rice milk, oat milk, nut milk and soya milk may be substituted.
- All processed foods (cakes, biscuits, sweets, ready meals, chocolate barsand so on). When buying bread, go for loaves made from whole grains and containing only 'good' fats, such as olive oil (ciabatta, for example).
- All fried foods.
- Sugar in all its forms (use honey instead).

Foods to be eaten as often as desired
- Vegetables and herbs.
- Fruit.
- Whole grains.
- Legumes.
- White fish.

Foods to be eaten in moderation
- Oily fish such as salmon and sardines.
- Seafood such as prawns and crab.
- Avocados.
- Nuts and seeds.
- Olives.

Occasional treats
Tea, coffee, alcohol – preferably wine, which contains antioxidants that are beneficial, but no more than two glasses a day, with at least two alcohol-free days per week.

Supplements for the Overcoming MS (OMS) diet

Take one omega-3 capsule on the days you don't eat oily fish. You should be able to get all the omega-6 you need from eating fruit and vegetables. If you are a vegetarian, you could take flaxseed oil instead, which contains both omega-3 and omega-6.

Cutting out meat may leave you short of vitamin B_{12}. You can take a daily vitamin B complex supplement or, if tests show your

B_{12} levels are very low, one 250 mcg or 1,000 mcg supplement once a week should be adequate.

You may wish to take 500 mg vitamin C twice a day (this is optional).

If you cannot get an adequate supply of vitamin D from sunlight, you will also need to take vitamin D supplements (see page 15).

Professor Jelinek advises avoiding multivitamins and antioxidants containing vitamins A and E as he feels that there is convincing evidence that they can be harmful if used in the long term.

7

The Wahls diet

When Terry Wahls, an American doctor, was first diagnosed with MS, she started taking disease-modifying drugs because – like many doctors in the UK and USA – she was unaware that any other form of therapy existed. However, by the time her disease had become progressive and she was regularly using a wheelchair, she had begun to trawl the internet to search for treatments that might be more successful than the drugs she was currently taking.

That was when she came across Ashton Embry's website, DIRECT-MS, and learnt for the first time that it was possible to use diet to treat MS. She looked at the scientific evidence provided on the website and decided it was reliable. She began to experiment with diet and supplements while continuing to research the body's biochemistry. Gradually she came to believe that the key to treating MS and other autoimmune diseases might lie with organisms called mitochondria, which are the body's powerhouse. They act like a battery, generating and releasing the energy that our cells need. Mitochondria produce a compound called ATP, which helps the body create proteins and antibodies. To do this, they need protection from toxins. They also need glucose, fat, oxygen, B vitamins, antioxidants, a selection of minerals, and co-enzyme Q10.

Without these nutrients, cells produce less energy, generate more free radicals and age prematurely. If you consume a diet high in sugar and starch, you are over 50 or you take regular medication, your mitochondria may be short of essential nutrients.

Dr Wahls went on to identify key nutrients needed to make healthy myelin, the nerve coating that is damaged in MS. These include more B vitamins, omega-3 fats and iodine. Also important are amino acids and sulphur, which are needed to make the neuro-transmitters that enable brain cells to talk to one another.

Having completed her research into the body's biochemistry, Dr Wahls concluded that what the body requires in order to heal is a diet that provides all the nutrients it needs from fresh, unadulterated plant and animal foods rather than supplements. She believes that real foods, rather than supplements, work in ways that we do not yet fully understand to meet the nutritional needs of every cell in our body. It may still be necessary, however, to take medication while the repair process continues.

This diet is a version of the Paleo diet – the sort of diet that hunter–gatherers ate thousands of years ago, before we grew crops and raised animals for consumption. It does, however, contain more nutrients than a standard Paleo diet. Where it differs markedly from all the other diets in this book is in its high fat content, obtained from oily fish, organic meat and poultry, coconut oil and avocados.

The diet has worked well for Dr Wahls, who has regained her health, can ride a bicycle once more and lectures regularly promoting her book, *The Wahls Protocol*. She and her team are now running clinical trials on patients with MS and other chronic diseases, using a combination of diet and exercise, and the University of Iowa is currently researching the Wahls diet. Like Professor Jelinek, Dr Wahls believes it is possible to recover from MS, although she admits that the diet doesn't work for everyone.

The diet

Fruit and vegetables

In order to obtain as wide a range of vitamins and minerals as possible, you need to consume 6–9 cups of vegetables and colourful fruit per day, depending on your size (a UK cup measure is based on a volume of 295 ml or 10 fl oz). This is made up of:

- 2–3 cups of green vegetables (chard, cress, parsley, lettuce, for example), which provide vitamins A, B, C and K;
- 2–3 cups of brightly coloured fruit and vegetables (such as kiwi fruit, red and yellow peppers, tomatoes, carrots), which provide antioxidants;
- 2–3 cups of sulphurous vegetables (such as cabbage, broccoli, cauliflower, onions, mushrooms), which nourish mitochondria and help eliminate toxins.

All fruit and vegetables should be organic and as fresh as possible, so they contain the maximum number of nutrients.

Proteins and fats

Eat between 260 g (9 oz) and 630 g (21 oz) protein every day in the form of grass-fed meat, wild game, organic free-range poultry, and line-caught fish. You should also eat about 340 g (12 oz) of organic meat (liver, kidney, etc.) per week to aid absorption of vitamin B_{12}. Meat contains amino acids, which cannot be manufactured by the body and must come from our diets.

You also need 1–2 cups of home-made bone broth every day, as well as some full-fat coconut milk. Bone broth contains glucosamine, which nourishes our bones and joints, as well as glutamine and amino acids, helping to heal a leaky gut.

Replace cow's milk with organic soya, rice, nut or coconut milk and use coconut oil for cooking, as it withstands high temperatures better than other plant oils.

NB You cannot follow this diet if you are a vegetarian, as meat provides the main natural source of amino acids and nutrients such as vitamin B_{12}.

Grains and legumes

Eat only wholemeal non-gluten grains such as brown rice, millet and quinoa, and organic legumes (peas, lentils, beans and chickpeas). Soak grains and legumes in water for 24 hours before cooking as they contain 'anti-nutrients' – phytates, which inhibit the absorption of vitamins and minerals; lections, which can increase inflammation in people with MS; and tripsin inhibitors, which block the ingestion of protein. NB The nightshade family (potatoes, tomatoes, peppers and aubergines) also contain lectins and may cause inflammation in some people with MS.

Other foods

Seaweed (a rich source of iodine) and fermented foods such as pickles and alcohol (small amounts of rum, wine or GF beer) are also allowed.

Foods to avoid

Avoid eggs, gluten, dairy products, sugar, vegetable oils and all processed foods, especially those containing hydrogenated and trans fats.

There are two further levels of this diet: the Wahls Paleo and the Wahls Paleo Plus, which are explained in detail in Dr Wahls' book, *The Wahls Protocol*. These progressively increase the fat intake and reduce carbohydrate intake to become eventually a ketogenic diet (high fat, no carbs). This is a very extreme diet, which is sometimes used by the medical profession as a treatment for severe epilepsy.

Warning The Wahls Paleo and the Wahls Paleo Plus diets should not be attempted except under medical supervision, as they could damage your liver or cause you to become dangerously underweight.

8

Getting started

Making cooking easier

You may have symptoms or disabilities that make preparing and cooking food difficult, so here are some tips to make cooking easier.

The basics

Read through the recipe and estimate how long it will take to prepare and cook it. Allow yourself ample time so you don't have to rush.

Before you start cooking, assemble all the equipment and ingredients you will need. Cut up any meat or vegetables; make stock; heat the oven; and grease and flour baking tins.

Do the preparation seated at the kitchen table. If you don't have one, see if you can borrow a perch stool from your local social services department; it enables you to take the weight off your feet while working at a counter.

If you have children or grandchildren, enlist their help in preparing the meal. Most children love cooking and enjoy getting involved.

Useful equipment

Food processor/blender

Many of these recipes use a food processor to cut out tiring mixing, beating and whisking. You don't need to buy a big, expensive one with lots of gadgets; a basic model that will mix, purée, slice and grate is all you need. If you won't be cooking for more than two people, you may find that a compact food processor with a 1.4-litre bowl will be quite adequate. Many food processors also come with a jug attachment, which can be used to make smoothies.

Microwave oven

My microwave gets used for far more than defrosting and heating up food. It helps speed up the cooking process in so many recipes and is invaluable for making granola and desserts such as Apricot and Banana Granola Crumble (page 128). You can cook vegetables quickly using a microwave steamer, and you can even use it to cook your Christmas pudding. As with food processors, the smallest, simplest ovens are often best. They're easier to use and there's less to go wrong.

Steamer

Steamers come in many different sizes and designs, from the economical bamboo bowl and lid that sits over a saucepan of boiling water to the self-contained electric steamer with several tiers that enables you to cook everything you need for a meal in one go, without using several pans full of boiling water.

Breadmaker

Many modern breadmakers have a special gluten-free (GF) programme for making gluten-free yeasted bread. However, there are now some GF soda bread mixes on the market, such as Orgran GF Bread Mix, that work well on the 'Rapid' programme of a standard breadmaker. These machines save you a lot of work. All you have to do is pour in the ingredients, press GO and come back when the bell rings at the end of the cycle. If you plan to make bread often, they are a good investment.

Tabletop fan

Cooking often generates a lot of heat, making the kitchen a very hostile environment for someone with MS. I overcome this problem by using a small tabletop fan.

Pots and pans

There is some evidence that aluminium saucepans are detrimental to health. Stainless steel pans don't carry these risks and are only slightly more expensive, and non-stick pans allow you to use less oil when browning meat and softening vegetables. Just take care not to scratch the coating with sharp knives or accidentally remove parts of it with abrasive cleaning agents. Buy pans with lids. You can boil water quicker and simmer food more successfully in a covered pan.

Measuring cups

To save fiddling with scales, I use measuring cups to measure out dry ingredients, and a microwaveable plastic measuring jug to measure liquids. If the liquid then has to be heated, the jug can go straight into the microwave. A standard UK measuring cup has a capacity of 295 ml (10 fl oz).

Knives

Make life easy for yourself: use the right knives for the job. You need a knife with a serrated edge for vegetables, and one with a smooth sharp blade for cutting meat.

Can opener and other tools

Look for the brands with thick plastic handles as they are easier to operate if you have a weak grip. If you cannot manage a manual can opener, buy a battery-powered wall-mounted model. Alternatively, look for cans with a ring pull, which are becoming increasingly common.

A garlic crusher, potato peeler, citrus juicer, pepper mill and pastry brush are also useful. These are all available from good kitchen shops or mail order from Lakeland (see Useful addresses).

Kitchen layout

Ideally your kitchen should be designed to minimize unnecessary movement, to eliminate the need to carry hot saucepans to and fro and to provide a convenient preparation area, preferably with a seat. You don't necessarily need a whole new kitchen – a little rearrangement may be all that is required.

Make sure all heavy items such as casserole dishes are on lower shelves for easy access, and store pots and pans and kitchen utensils adjacent to the cooker. If you have a dishwasher, this should be near the sink, as should the waste bin.

In a larger kitchen, a table in the middle of the room can serve as a preparation area, a dinner table and a convenient surface on which to place objects you wish to move across the room. This helps to prevent broken plates and spillages.

If you use a wheelchair, you will need expert advice on how to adapt your kitchen to suit your needs. Again, your local social services department should be able to advise you and should know of any grants available to help you finance the work.

Food safety

If you are unused to cooking, you may be unaware of the few simple rules that could help protect you against food poisoning. Infections are easy to prevent, so why take risks?

- Always wash your hands thoroughly before cooking and remove any rings.
- Throw out any foods in your fridge or larder that have passed their 'use by' or 'best before' dates, especially if they are protein foods, such as eggs or meat.
- Use separate chopping boards for meat and vegetables or chop the vegetables first. This prevents cross-contamination from the meat. Scrub boards well after each use.
- Defrost all meat, fish and poultry thoroughly before cooking and do not refreeze any food once it has been defrosted.
- Meat, fish and poultry must be cooked right through or, if already cooked, thoroughly reheated in order to kill all bacteria. Be particularly careful with barbecued food; even when it is burnt on the outside, it may still be raw inside.
- Don't eat raw eggs – in desserts made from uncooked egg whites, for example.

Shopping for food

When you embark on one of the diets in this book, you may find you have to change your shopping habits. Organization is essential to ensure that you always have a supply of food available to suit your needs. Before you shop, draw up a menu list for the week ahead, and check the contents of your larder and fridge so you can work out a detailed shopping list.

If you have a butcher, greengrocer or fishmonger nearby, make the most of them. A good butcher should be able to tell you exactly where the meat came from and whether it is organic, grass-fed or corn-fed. The butcher can also mince or cube meat for you, and fishmongers can fillet fish, which will make life much easier. Local shopkeepers can also sell you small quantities of food, whereas much supermarket meat or fish is sold in big packs aimed at families. Small shopkeepers are eager to help regular customers, so you may find they will even deliver your food for you.

Don't overlook markets as they are often a good source of locally grown fruit and vegetables, some of which may be organic. An increasing number of organic farms supply boxes of fruit and vegetables. You can get a list from the Soil Association (see Useful addresses).

Supermarkets now cater for those with special dietary needs, as well as supplying a range of foods with less fat and sugar. The larger supermarkets have in-store bakeries, butchers, fishmongers and delicatessens, and it's worth using these for their fresh, good-quality food rather than buying packaged meat, chicken and bread that will almost certainly be cheaper but less nutritious. More and more supermarkets now offer online ordering and home delivery – time-consuming perhaps the first time you do it, but easier and well worth it once you learn your way around the virtual store. On supermarket websites you can also find a list of ingredients for every product they sell – invaluable if you need to avoid certain foods.

For anyone on a special diet, health food shops are a godsend. I regularly buy rice or almond milk, wholegrain pasta, brown rice, pulses and supplements from my local family-run health food shop and they deliver my order once a fortnight. There are now also many mail order companies offering a range of foods to suit special diets (see Useful addresses).

Many people ask if a special diet will cost more. The short answer is yes, it probably will, although it really depends what you spent on food before. The cheapest food you can buy is junk food – crisps, chocolate bars, burgers – which is why so many people on low incomes are overweight and unhealthy. You generally do have to pay more for good quality fresh food. However, if you do not require specialist food such as gluten-free bread, and you are used to living on microwave meals and takeaways, you may actually save money by cooking all your meals from scratch. Buying food that is in season instead of produce flown in from abroad will save you money and will also, as a bonus, benefit the environment. Table 3.1 (page 34) shows when fruits and vegetables are in season.

Food labelling

EU food labelling regulations that came into force in December 2014 can help you understand whether or not a particular food will meet your needs.

Colour-coded nutritional information on the food's packaging will tell you if the item has low, medium or high levels of fat, saturated fat, salt and sugar. Red indicates high levels; amber equals medium levels; and green shows low levels. The more green on the label, the healthier the food.

Other useful symbols to look out for are the:

- Soil Association logo, which guarantees the food is organic;
- Marine Stewardship Council (MSC) label, which indicates the fish comes from a sustainable source;
- Freedom Foods label, which indicates the animals have been reared to strict welfare standards, but does not mean the food is organic;
- Red Tractor for Assured Food Standards, which appears on meat products and guarantees the animal was reared in Britain, but is not a quality guarantee;
- Crossed Grain symbol, which guarantees the food is gluten-free.

If any of the 14 most common allergens are present in a food (such as milk, gluten, peanuts), they must be clearly identified in the ingredients list, often in bold type. Note that wheat from which the gluten has been removed is classified as 'gluten-free', so if you want to avoid wheat altogether, go for 'wheat- and gluten-free'.

E numbers, colours, preservatives, flavourings and sweeteners must also be listed on the packet. Any product with a long list of additives is best avoided if you have MS.

Eating out

With a bit of advance planning, there is no reason why your special diet should prevent you enjoying a meal out with friends and family. Phone the restaurant in advance and explain what your requirements are to either the chef or the manager. If there's nothing on the menu to suit you, maybe an existing dish can be adapted. More and more restaurants are now becoming aware of the need to cater for customers' special dietary needs, and several UK restaurant chains, such as Ask, Frankie and Benny's, Hard Rock Café and Carluccio's, now provide some GF menu options. If you are disabled, don't forget to check accessibility and toilet facilities at the same time you check the food.

Buy a tailor-made dietary alert card from <www.dietarycard. co.uk> and hand it to the waiter. The card will list those foods you can eat and those you wish to avoid, and you can even get foreign language versions to use when travelling abroad.

If you are on a more restricted diet, a book you may find helpful is *Let's Eat Out! Your passport to living gluten and allergy free* by Kim Koeller and Robert La France (R. and R. Publishing, 2005). Although the book was originally published more than ten years ago, much of the material is still relevant. Despite it being an American publication, this book is of use to anyone with food intolerances, wherever you live. It helps you select menu items from seven different national cuisines; lists global airlines with special meal options; and includes useful multilingual phrases needed when discussing food. The allergens covered include corn, dairy, wheat, gluten, nuts, soya and eggs. It is available from Amazon and other booksellers.

Holidays

If you are holidaying in the UK, you may be better off in self-catering accommodation where you have control over what you eat, and if you travel by car you can take a good supply of essential ingredients. It's probably not a good idea to stay anywhere too remote, where getting hold of fresh food or speciality items may be a problem. It can be useful to contact the local tourist information centre in advance to check the location of the nearest supermarket and health food shop.

Holiday camps usually have an on-site shop but they rarely carry a good supply of fresh fruit and vegetables. Cooking equipment is usually pretty basic too, so remember to pack essential implements such as a good sharp knife for slicing vegetables and a can opener. Some holiday apartments will provide you with a box of groceries of your choice on arrival, which is useful if you are travelling by public transport and can't take much food with you.

Case studies

Anna

I first experienced symptoms in the summer of 2011. I had pins and needles in my feet that started working up my legs until they reached my hips, and sometimes I woke in the night with a completely numb arm.

My doctor arranged for me to have blood tests, which all came back clear. When I was still having strange sensations a few weeks later, I was referred to a neurologist, who arranged for me to have an MRI scan. By now my legs felt tired and heavy when I was walking up the stairs, and my left thigh was a few centimetres thinner than my right thigh.

The first scan was inconclusive, but a further MRI scan in April 2012 showed two old lesions plus another active lesion. The neurologist confirmed that the most likely diagnosis was MS, but wanted to do further tests to be certain.

That was when I began researching MS. I bought *Overcoming Multiple Sclerosis* and read how diet and lifestyle changes had had a positive impact on Professor Jelinek's MS. I liked the fact it was based on solid scientific research and the idea of being able to do something myself to deal with the disease. It seemed the earlier I changed my diet, the more positive the outcome was likely to be. Taking control of the situation made me feel psychologically better.

By the time I had the last tests, I was experiencing fresh symptoms. I made the decision there and then to start the diet. In October 2012 I finally received a definitive diagnosis of relapsing–remitting MS. I was offered a choice of disease-modifying drugs and I chose Copaxone. Although I was relieved to have a diagnosis at last, I was also fearful for the future.

I now follow the OMS programme, which includes diet, exercise and meditation. I eat a plant-based wholefood diet supplemented with seafood, but I do not eat oily fish. My diet is dairy-free and low in saturated fat. I take vitamin D, vitamin B and a tablespoon of flaxseed oil on the days I don't eat fish.

Although the diet forbids meat and egg yolks, I do occasionally eat lean turkey breast and a whole egg. As gluten is allowed, I still eat bread although I try not to eat too much. As I have a naturally small build, I have to be careful not to become too underweight. I have blood tests on a yearly basis and they have shown that my vitamin, folate and iron levels are all still fine.

My old diet contained a lot of foods high in saturated fat, such as cheese, butter and red meat. I drank numerous cups of tea and coffee every day and ate chocolate bars or a piece of cake for energy, and few of my meals were made from scratch. I rarely ate fish. It was a major change to my lifestyle to eat this new way, and it took about a month to completely change to the OMS diet.

The new diet has made a difference to my health. I now have more energy and, when I jog, I can run faster and feel less out of breath. I play tennis three times a week and can comfortably run 5 km in less than 30 minutes.

I am very pleased that an MRI scan in October 2014 showed no active lesions and no new ones. I believe that any intermittent symptoms I have are from the lesions that are already there, but my MS symptoms do return temporarily if I get a virus or infection.

My advice for anyone thinking of going down the dietary route is to ensure you make time to plan meals, shop and prepare the food, because it is tempting to stray from the diet if you are tired and do not have the right foods in the house. Going out for meals with friends can be tricky, so it is worth explaining the diet to them. However, whatever the difficulties, I would never return to how I ate before. I no longer crave cakes and chocolate bars, and making food from scratch has allowed me to discover new recipes and new flavours.

What surprises me is how little the neurologists and MS nurses I meet know about the diet I am on. They may not be allowed to recommend diet therapy, but I feel they should read up on the work of Dr Swank, Professor Jelinek and Dr Wahls so they are aware of what patients may be trying.

Beth

My MS was diagnosed nearly 20 years ago, although I had my first symptoms a couple of years before that. I have had some really nasty relapses but am lucky to have had long periods between relapses and to have made a good recovery every time.

My last major relapse was about seven and a half years ago. At that stage I wasn't fully following the Overcoming MS diet, but it was probably that relapse that forced me into making the final changes to comply more rigidly with the diet. Almost exactly a year later I had a very minor relapse and that was the first time I had ever qualified for disease-modifying drugs. I started on Copaxone nearly six years ago and have recently changed to using Tecfidera. I haven't had any relapses since starting on medication, but also during that time I have become much more disciplined about the OMS diet, so it's quite difficult to separate the two influences.

I have been following all of the OMS recommendations – diet, exercise, vitamin D, meditation – for about seven years now. It appealed to me because George Jelinek was a doctor and had approached the problem in a scientific way, but also because I was already a vegetarian (although not a very healthy one!) and had never really liked dairy products. Although it wasn't too far from my existing diet I had to make quite a lot of changes to my eating habits, and I implemented these gradually over a period of about three years.

I have been vegetarian for all of my adult life, and I used to eat quite a lot of processed foods such as quiche, chips and biscuits, and not much fruit and vegetables. I also ate milk, cheese and yogurt and would snack on chocolate and crisps, so it was quite a big change to introduce fish and stop the dairy products. I didn't really miss the dairy at all and to this day have barely used any substitutes, apart from the occasional soya yogurt.

I mainly drink water, although I have a herbal tea from time to time, I don't drink tea or coffee so I don't need any milk for drinks and I've found that quite easy to adjust to. I no longer cook with oil; instead I 'dry fry' foods or boil or steam them, and I always inspect the labels on food packets to see what they contain. I am very disciplined with my saturated fat intake and aim to stay below 10 mg per day. I have an app on my phone into which I put my food for the day, and it gives me a saturated fat count, as well as other dietary information.

Because I've been following the diet for a long time now, I no longer have to think too much about which foods to eat and which to avoid, but I do check any new foods or meals carefully. I like the variety of meals that are available on the diet and I find it very easy to stick to. It's a much healthier diet than I used to have. It can be tricky when eating out, but people are usually quite accommodating, especially if I phone ahead and discuss my dietary requirements with the restaurant. It can be hard to change food habits, but it's definitely possible if you have the right motivation, and seeing myself remaining well is the best motivation I could wish for.

At the moment I am fit and well with no real MS symptoms most of the time. I have a busy family life and a part-time job. I regularly exercise and took up running about five years ago, and in that time I have done 12 half marathons. I also regularly do Pilates and go to the gym.

I don't know what it is that is keeping me well – whether it is the OMS lifestyle, medication or just luck – but I feel the OMS recommendations are healthy and am going to continue with them. When I talk about my diet I can sound a bit of a 'weirdo', but I can live with that and I have no intention of changing what I do. In fact, I think other people respect my choices, and friends will often say that they couldn't do it themselves but they admire me for sticking to it.

Paula

When I was diagnosed with MS in 2001, it was a massive shock. I had previously led a very busy and active life, travelling and working around the world. I had also played squash at a national level. After my diagnosis I began to study diet. I started out on the Overcoming MS diet and was pretty stable. However, recently I discovered *The Wahls Protocol* and am now eating something more like a Paleo diet.

I am strict about what I eat. I start the morning with a green smoothie, with added lecithin and a green spirolina powder, followed by sausages, salmon or egg, mushrooms and tomato.

All the fish and meat I eat is organic and grass-fed or wild. I never eat farmed meat or fish. I eat calf's liver once or twice a week and make bone stock from organic beef bones. All the fruit and vegetables I eat are also fresh and organic.

I eat very little potatoes and rice, and no gluten at all. I don't bother with gluten-free products as they are full of other nasties! Instead I make my own gluten-free snack: lemon and almond biscotti (almond flour, organic honey and organic lemon). I've avoided dairy too ever since an MRI scan showed one of my sinuses was blocked. I had a sinus operation a few years ago and have not touched dairy since.

Apart from one cup of espresso and one cup of fennel tea every day and a small amount of red wine on three nights a week, I only drink water.

I stopped taking Copaxone in 2007 and I haven't taken any drugs since. I do take some supplements, though: 1,000 mg vitamin C, 5,000 iu vitamin D, calcium, magnesium, zinc and a multivitamin, plus a daily probiotic. I saw a new neurologist recently and he could not believe how well I was doing. He tried to persuade me to go back on disease-modifying drugs, but I said no.

My main symptoms are concentration and memory problems and cognitive issues, plus a left leg that tingles all the time. However, my symptoms are well under control and I am honestly feeling a big improvement since starting the Wahls diet in May 2015, more than I did on the Overcoming MS diet. There is a theory that different blood groups should eat different types of food. My blood type is O (caveman and meat eater, apparently), so the Wahls diet probably makes more sense for me. I believe the addition of meat has dramatically helped with fatigue. I can now go mountain-biking several times a week without suffering serious fatigue, and the tingling in my leg is reducing slightly. The green smoothies, too, have helped with memory and concentration. I also do yoga and meditation regularly, and have a massage at least once a week.

David

I have been following the Wahls diet for seven years now and started to notice improvements in my health almost immediately.

Before I started the diet, my throat, tongue and sinuses were affected and my mouth had begun to sag on one side, so that I had lost my smile. I had also lost sensation in my hands and feet, had a permanent knot in my upper back and couldn't rotate my arms freely.

My diet is now dairy-free, gluten-free and sugar-free, and I take the supplements recommended by Dr Wahls: fish oil, vitamin D_3 tablets, brewer's yeast tablets and co-enzyme Q10. I also add seaweed to my evening meal. The only pain relief I take now is paracetamol.

The diet seems to work by flooding a particular part of the body with increased blood supply and heat – a sort of 'healthy healing inflammation'. It can be quite painful and is not for the faint-hearted. No pain, no gain, as they say. It feels as if, when a part of your body is actively under repair, the nerves 'go on holiday' while they are in the process of healing.

At the moment, it feels as though the disease is receding as sensation is slowly returning to my hands and feet – the parts of my body most badly affected by the MS. The swelling I had around my knees has gone down by about 90 per cent, and the knot in my shoulders has disappeared. I am much more comfortable at night and, best of all, I can smile again!

The diet has also helped my psoriasis (another autoimmune disease), which I had on various parts of my body. Now I only have some patches on my legs and it has almost disappeared from my scalp.

Rikki

Although I was diagnosed in 2003, I chose to put my head in the sand about the problem for many years. However in 2013, despite me being on Avonex, my balance and coordination began to deteriorate, which limited the distance I could walk. I was also experiencing bladder urgency and eye pain. That was when I decided I had to do something. After a lot of research (a lot of it conflicting) I decided to go with the Overcoming MS diet.

Since then, I have been following the eating plan, and taking flaxseed oil and vitamin D_3 supplements. I am walking further and I have more energy than I did two years ago, and my bladder problems and eye pain have almost disappeared. Improvements are subtle, and it does require a lot of determination to stick to the diet, but there are lots of encouraging stories on the Overcoming MS website to spur me on.

After being on Avonex for 11 years I stopped it about four months ago as I had developed side effects. I have more energy since coming off the drug, and I now think it did me more harm than good. I am still not great but I am much better than I was, and Professor Jelinek does say it can take around three to five years for improvements to be noticed.

I have no reservations about recommending the OMS approach to anyone with MS. It is healthy eating, and there is nothing in it that can do anybody any harm.

Vera
I was diagnosed with MS in 2001. At this point I was told that drugs would be available but I wasn't 'bad enough' to need them. Some years later I started taking LDN, which I had to pay for privately. I took it for several years and it improved my mood and made me more optimistic, but I've never taken any other drugs for MS.

I soon discovered Ashton Embry and began the Best Bet diet in 2003. Since then I have tried a lot of diets, not all of them for MS. They all seemed to help for a while, which I now put down to the placebo effect, since I have continued to slowly decline. However, I have only had one relapse, which occurred after a period of enormous stress.

In 2012 I tried the Overcoming MS diet for nine months, but it didn't help me at all and I hated taking all the fish oil supplements. Later that year I started the Wahls diet, which is the only diet that has had an immediate and lasting effect on me. After only three days I felt great. My fatigue disappeared and walking improved. I got used to being awake all day, doing swimming and Pilates classes, and walking the dog. After I'd been on the Wahls diet for about two months, I felt so good that I stopped taking the LDN. I was also able to reduce the dose of another drug, Thyroxine, which I have been taking for over 20 years for an underactive thyroid.

I had been working from Terry Wahls' *Minding My Mitochondria* (TZ Press, second edition, 2010), which suggested a very low-calorie diet. Unfortunately I couldn't keep up the diet because I lost too much weight and wasn't eating enough in the winter to sustain me. I then started to eat porridge every day and added more good fats such as olive oil, hemp oil and duck fat, and eventually my weight stabilized. By the following winter my diet was grain-free and I felt fine.

When Terry Wahls' book *The Wahls Protocol* came out in 2015, I was amazed to see she was now following a very similar diet to me. I still have plenty of energy and no real fatigue, but my walking has continued to decline, so I'm still looking for solutions. I've never felt quite so good as I did in those first three months after starting the Wahls diet.

Part 3
THE RECIPES

Guidance on following the recipes

Where 'milk' is specified, use whichever milk is recommended for the diet you are following.

Where 'yogurt' is specified, this means natural unflavoured bio-yogurt made from cow's milk for the healthy eating diet, low-fat diet and vegetarian diet, soya yogurt for the vegan diet and coconut yogurt for the Wahls diet.

Where 'flour' is specified, use a good quality unbleached white flour or wholemeal flour for the healthy eating diet, low-fat diet, Overcoming MS diet, vegetarian and vegan diet, and a wholegrain gluten-free flour such as rice flour for the Best Bet diet and Wahls diet, or if you cannot tolerate wheat or gluten.

Abbreviations

HED	healthy eating diet
LFD	low-fat diet
BBD	Best Bet diet
OMSD	Overcoming MS diet
WD	Wahls diet
VEG	vegetarian diet
VG	vegan diet

1 tsp = 1 teaspoon
1 dsp = 1 dessertspoon
1 tbsp = 1 tablespoon
1 cup = 295 ml (10 fl oz)

Oven temperatures

°C	°F	Gas mark
140 °C	275 °F	1
150 °C	300 °F	2
160 °C	325 °F	3
180 °C	350 °F	4
190 °C	375 °F	5
200 °C	400 °F	6
220 °C	425 °F	7
230 °C	450 °F	8

Breakfasts

Porridge

HED LFD OMSD VEG VG (Serves 1)

½ cup porridge oats
1 cup milk of choice
½ cup water

Put the oats and liquids in a saucepan and bring to the boil. Turn down heat and simmer, stirring until mixture has thickened.

If cooking in the microwave, use only ½ cup water and ½ cup milk. Put water, milk and oats in a glass bowl or microwave saucepan and cook on high for 1 minute. Stir well, then cook on high for a further minute. Serve with added milk and fresh fruit, such as blueberries, or dried fruit, such as raisins or sultanas.

Porridge

BBD (Serves 1)

¼ cup rice or buckwheat flakes
¼ cup millet flakes
½ cup water
½ cup rice milk

Put all ingredients in a saucepan and bring to boil. Simmer, stirring, for about 5 minutes until mixture has thickened.

Granola

HED LFD OMSD VEG VG (Serves 5)

This crunchy muesli will keep in the fridge for a week. Serve with fresh fruit and your milk of choice.

2 cups porridge oats
2 dsp runny honey
2 dsp olive oil
¼ cup sesame seeds
¼ cup sunflower seeds
¼ cup chia seeds
¼ cup chopped nuts
½ cup dried fruit such as raisins or currants

Put the oats, honey and oil in a large microwaveable bowl. Mix well. Cook, uncovered, on high in the microwave for 2 minutes. Stir, then cook on high for another 2 minutes. Leave to cool, then mix in seeds, nuts and dried fruit.

Granola

BBD (Serves 5)

As above, but replace porridge oats with a mixture of rice flakes and buckwheat flakes.

Granola

WD (Serves 5)

As above, but replace oats with a mixture of rice flakes and buckwheat flakes.

Replace olive oil with coconut oil and add ¼ cup coconut flakes with the nuts and seeds. Serve with nut milk or coconut milk.

Granola Delight

HED LFD WD VEG VG (Serves 1)

Place fruit such as berries, a diced kiwi fruit or a sliced banana in a large dessert bowl and cover with a cup of unsweetened yogurt. Sprinkle 4 dsp granola over and drizzle a little honey on top.

Marinated Spiced Fruit

HED LFD BBD OMSD WD VEG VG (Serves 1)

4 dried apricots
4 stoned dried prunes
4 dried figs
½ cup orange juice
½ tsp ground cinnamon

Soak fruit and spice in juice overnight. Serve topped with yogurt or Cashew Nut Cream (page 129).

Smoothies

Smoothies are a quick and easy way to boost your nutrient intake. Green smoothies, in which vegetables are added to the basic fruit mixture, are a staple of the Wahls diet. In each case, place all ingredients in a blender and whizz until smooth.

Fruit Smoothie

HED LFD BBD OMSD WD VEG VG (Serves 1)

1 small banana, quartered
1 cup strawberries, blackberries or blueberries
½ cup milk of choice

Green Smoothie

HED LFD BBD OMSD WD VEG VG (Serves 1)

1 apple, peeled, cored and cut into chunks
1 ripe avocado, peeled, stoned and cut into chunks
large handful baby spinach or kale
150 ml (¼ pt) water

Soups, dips and pâtés

Unless indicated otherwise, all soups can be frozen.

If you are on the Best Bet diet, all vegetable stock for soups should be made with yeast-free granules or stock cubes.

If you are following the Wahls diet, replace olive oil with coconut oil and vegetable stock with home-made Bone Broth (see page 135 for recipe).

Middle Eastern Lentil Soup

HED LFD OMSD VEG VG (Serves 2)

1 small leek, chopped
1 dsp olive oil
2 level tsp ground cumin
1 garlic clove, crushed, or 1 tsp garlic purée
1 large carrot, peeled and sliced
2 celery sticks, sliced
600 ml (1 pt) vegetable stock
60 g (2 oz) red lentils
1 dsp tomato purée
salt and black pepper

Soften leek in oil in a large pan over a low heat for a few minutes.

Add cumin and garlic and stir for 1 minute. Add vegetables, stock, lentils and tomato purée. Bring to boil. Cover pan, turn down heat and simmer for 30 minutes.

Purée in food processor. Reheat in saucepan, adding a little hot water if mixture is too thick. Season to taste with salt and black pepper.

Sweet Potato and Coriander Soup

HED LFD BBD OMSD WD VEG VG (Serves 2)

1 medium leek, sliced
1 dsp olive oil
1 large carrot, peeled and sliced
1 sweet potato, about 150 mm (6 in) long, peeled and sliced
¼ tsp mild chilli powder
½ tsp ground cumin
600 ml (1 pt) vegetable stock
½ pack fresh coriander, leaves roughly chopped
salt and black pepper

Soften leek in oil in a saucepan over a low heat for 5 minutes. Add carrot, sweet potato and spices and stir for 1 minute. Add stock and bring mixture to boil. Turn down heat, cover pan and simmer for 15 minutes. Put soup in processor with fresh coriander. Purée, season with salt and black pepper and reheat.

Herbs

Using herbs in cooking not only adds subtle flavours to the food you eat but benefits your health, too.

Parsley is particularly good for you as it is packed with vitamin C. It also contains vitamins A and B and large amounts of iron, plus calcium and magnesium, and it helps your body to digest food.

Thyme and rosemary have health-giving properties as they are full of antioxidants, and rosemary tea can help improve memory and concentration and lift depression.

Leek and Potato Soup

HED LFD OMSD BBD WD VEG VG (Serves 2)

2 celery sticks, sliced
1 large garlic clove, crushed
1 tbsp olive oil
1 leek, sliced
1 carrot, peeled and sliced
1 medium potato, peeled and cut into chunks
600 ml (1 pt) vegetable stock
handful fresh parsley, chopped
salt and black pepper

Soften celery and garlic in oil in a saucepan on a low heat for 5 minutes. Add all the other ingredients, apart from the parsley. Bring pan to boil, turn down heat and simmer, covered, for 20 minutes. Add parsley and season with salt and black pepper. For a smooth soup, purée in food processor before serving.

Cock-a-leekie Soup

HED LFD BBD WD (Serves 2)

Add a large handful of cooked chicken to Leek and Potato Soup (see above) for last 5 minutes of cooking.

Broccoli and Courgette Soup

HED LFD BBD OMSD VEG VG (Serves 2)

1 large leek, sliced
1 dsp olive oil
1 garlic clove, crushed
1 medium courgette, sliced
2 tsp ground coriander
600 ml (1 pt) vegetable stock
1 medium head broccoli, divided into florets
1 dsp cornflour mixed with 1 dsp water
salt and black pepper

In a large pan, soften leek in oil over a low heat for a few minutes. Add garlic, courgette and coriander and mix well. Add stock, broccoli and cornflour and bring to the boil. Turn down heat and simmer, covered, for 10 minutes. Purée in a food processor, season well with salt and black pepper and reheat.

Fish Soup

HED LFD BBD OMSD WD (Serves 1)

1 celery stick, sliced
½ red pepper, deseeded and sliced
½ small courgette, sliced
1 garlic clove, crushed
1 dsp olive oil
1 dsp flour
300 ml (½ pt) fish stock
1 fillet white fish (about 115 g or 4 oz), cut into bite-sized pieces
⅓ cup sweetcorn
1 tbsp fresh parsley, chopped
a few cooked prawns

Soften celery, pepper, courgette and garlic in oil over a low heat for 5 minutes. Mix in flour, then add stock, fish and sweetcorn. Bring to boil, lower heat and simmer, covered, for 10 minutes. Stir in parsley and prawns and heat through. Season with salt if required. Do not freeze the soup if you used frozen fish and prawns to make it.

Minestrone Soup

HED LFD OMSD VEG VG (Serves 4)

This classic Italian soup is ideal for a family meal. Keep a check on the pasta so it doesn't become mushy.

1 leek, chopped
2 celery sticks, chopped
2 large garlic cloves, crushed, or 2 tsp garlic purée
1 tbsp olive oil
2 dsp rice flour
2 medium carrots, peeled and sliced
725 ml (1¼ pt) vegetable stock
400-g (14-oz) tin chopped tomatoes
1 tsp Italian herb seasoning
400-g (14-oz) tin kidney beans, drained and well rinsed
½ cup frozen green beans
½ cup pasta tubes
2 large green cabbage leaves, shredded
salt and black pepper

Soften leek, celery and garlic in oil over a low heat for a few minutes. Mix in rice flour. Add carrots, stock, tomatoes and herbs. Bring to boil and simmer, covered, for 10 minutes.

Add kidney beans, green beans, pasta and cabbage. Bring back to boil, turn down heat and simmer, covered, for another 10 minutes until the pasta is just cooked. Season well with salt and black pepper before serving.

Hummus

HED LFD OMSD VEG VG (Serves 4)

1 large (400-g) can chickpeas, drained and well rinsed
2 garlic cloves, crushed
2 tbsp tahini paste
juice of 1 lemon
1 tbsp olive oil
1 tbsp water
salt and black pepper
1 tsp paprika

Ensure you've removed all the pips from the lemon juice, then blend everything together in a food processor. If mixture is too thick, add another tablespoon of water and blend again. Sprinkle with paprika before serving.

Salmon Pâté

HED LFD (Serves 1)

4 spring onions, finely chopped
1 tsp olive oil
210-g (7-oz) tin salmon chunks
2 level tbsp natural yogurt
1 tbsp fresh parsley, chopped
1 tsp paprika
salt and black pepper

Put spring onions and oil in a glass bowl and microwave on medium high for 30 seconds. Drain salmon and put in processor with spring onions and oil. Add yogurt, parsley and paprika and season with salt and black pepper. Blend until smooth.

Sardine Pâté

HED LFD OMSD BBD (Serves 1)

1 tin sardines, drained
1 dsp olive oil
1 dsp lemon juice
1 tsp garlic purée
1 tbsp fresh parsley, chopped
black pepper

Put ingredients in food processor and whizz until smooth.

Guacamole

HED LFD OMSD BBD WD VEG VG (Serves 2)

2 avocados, peeled, stoned and chopped
juice of 1 lime
½ tsp salt
2 spring onions, thinly sliced
2 tbsp fresh coriander, chopped
4 cherry tomatoes, chopped
1 garlic clove, crushed
pinch cayenne pepper
2 dsp extra virgin olive oil

Mix all ingredients together in a bowl or, for a smoother result, whizz in a food processor.

Vegetables and whole grains

Vegetables form an important part of all the diets in this book. Here's how to prepare and cook them so that their all-important nutrients are not lost in the process.

- **Potatoes** Leaving the peel on potatoes when you cook them enables you to benefit from the vitamin C that is just underneath the skin.
- **Baked potatoes** Allow 1 large potato per person. Heat oven to 220 °C (425 °F, gas mark 7). Scrub the potato well and make a large cross on the top and bottom with a sharp knife (this prevents the potato bursting out of its skin as it heats up). Cook on high in the microwave for 2 minutes, then turn over and cook for a further 2 minutes. Remove from microwave, place on a baking tray and cook for 20 minutes in the oven to crisp up the skin. If cooking more than one potato at once, increase time in microwave.

Accompaniments for Baked Potatoes

HED

- A small tin of tuna or salmon mixed with some low-fat mayonnaise and chopped fresh parsley.
- Grated low-fat Cheddar cheese.

LFD

- Cottage cheese mixed with chopped fresh chives and a pinch of paprika.
- Chopped cooked chicken mixed with natural yogurt and 1 tsp mustard.

BBD

- Chopped cooked chicken or turkey mixed with chopped tomato and cucumber and fresh coriander in an oil and lemon dressing.
- Tinned tuna or salmon with 2 tbsp passata, heated in the microwave.

OMSD

- Cooked prawns in yogurt dressing with chopped fresh parsley.
- Guacamole.

Potato Wedges

HED LFD BBD OMSD VEG VG (Serves 2)

Preheat oven to 220 °C (425 °F, gas mark 7). Scrub 450 g (1 lb) medium-sized potatoes and cut each in half lengthways, then in half again to form a wedge shape. Put the wedges on an oiled baking tray and brush with a small amount of oil. Season with salt and black pepper and bake in the preheated oven for about 45 minutes. They should be crisp and browned on the outside and soft inside.

Sweet Potato Wedges

HED LFD BBD OMSD VEG VG (Serves 2)

Sweet potatoes, which contain twice as much fibre and calcium and far more vitamin A than ordinary potatoes, can be cooked in the same way as Potato Wedges (see above, using same quantities). If they are old and gnarled, however, they may need to be peeled first.

Indian Spiced Wedges

HED LFD BBD OMSD VEG VG (Serves 2)

Marinade
1 tsp ground cumin
1 tsp ground coriander
½ tsp salt
½ tsp mild chilli powder
1 tbsp olive oil

Mix all ingredients together. Both potato and sweet potato wedges can be coated in this marinade, then baked as in the Potato Wedges recipe (see above).

Dark-green leafy vegetables

Spring greens and cabbage

Discard any discoloured and damaged leaves and, using a knife with a serrated edge, cut off the woody base. Chop into small pieces, place in a sieve and rinse well. Cook in a steamer for 5 or 6 minutes. Take care not to overcook them.

Spinach

One bag of baby spinach leaves will serve 3–4 people.

Remove leaves from bag and put in a large sieve. Rinse well, then put them, still wet, into a large saucepan. Don't add any extra water. Cover pan and cook leaves over a low heat for 4 minutes until they become a homogenous dark green mass. Drain before serving.

Broccoli and cauliflower

One head of broccoli or one medium cauliflower is enough for 4 people. Cut off the thick base and any outer leaves and divide the remainder into individual florets. Broccoli and cauliflower should be steamed for about 6 or 7 minutes.

The onion family

Red onions, brown onions, spring onions, leeks and garlic are all part of the onion family and have a distinctive sharp taste. Spring onions and leeks are easier to prepare than brown onions, and less likely to cause watery eyes. However, in many cases these vegetables are interchangeable, so use whatever is easiest for you.

If you find preparing garlic fiddly, you can substitute garlic purée (available in tubes) or chopped garlic in oil (in jars). Processed garlic doesn't have the same health-giving properties as fresh garlic, but the result is perfectly acceptable.

Onions

Small red onions have a milder taste than the larger brown onions and can be eaten raw in salads. To prepare an onion, place it on chopping board and, using a really sharp knife, cut off the hard base and top, which may have green shoots. Now cut it in half vertically and peel off the papery outer leaves. Turn one half of the onion on its side and slice thinly from one side to the other, then turn it through 90 degrees and slice again from side to side. Repeat with the other half. The onion should now be in small pieces.

Leeks

Leeks often have soil in between the layers, so need to be cleaned thoroughly. Cut off most of the thick green tops of the leaves. Then slice vertically down through the centre of the leek and pull the layers gently apart. Hold under running water and rinse well to remove any dirt. Pull off the thick outer leaf and cut away the root section. Last, cut the whole thing in half lengthways and slice thinly.

Garlic

Start by separating out a single clove of garlic from the bulb. Using a sharp knife, cut off the pointed tip and the hard base. Tease off the papery outer covering and place clove in a garlic crusher. Press down hard and shreds of garlic will appear through the holes and can be scraped off with a knife.

Garlic

As well as adding flavour to food, garlic has many health benefits. Its principal active ingredient is allicin, which helps regulate cholesterol levels and also reduces the stickiness of blood platelets, so assisting blood flow. Garlic has antibacterial properties, too, and can help treat infections and boost immunity.

Eating garlic with your food encourages the body to absorb less fat, so it is particularly helpful if you are on a low-fat diet. Eat it raw for maximum health benefit. To prevent 'garlic breath', eat it with fresh parsley. Odourless garlic supplements are also available.

Recipes for vegetables

Roasted Summer Vegetables

HED LFD BBD OMSD VEG VG (Serves 2)

Roasting brings out the sweetness in vegetables such as onion and peppers.

1 medium onion, peeled and quartered
1 medium courgette, cut into 2.5-cm (1-in) sections
1 red pepper, deseeded and quartered
1 green pepper, deseeded and quartered
2 large tomatoes, halved
1 dsp olive oil
1 large garlic clove, crushed, or 1 tsp garlic purée
salt and black pepper

Preheat oven to 200 °C (400 °F, gas mark 6). Place prepared vegetables in an oiled baking dish. Mix oil and garlic and brush over vegetables. Season well with salt and black pepper. Cook in the preheated oven for about 45 minutes, until vegetables are soft and beginning to brown.

Oven-roasted Vegetables with Pasta

HED LFD OMSD BBD (Serves 2)

Add either a handful of cashew nuts or a can of drained anchovies to the vegetables in the previous recipe for the last 5 minutes of cooking and serve with pasta for a satisfying main dish.

Roasted Winter Vegetables

HED LFD BBD OMSD VEG VG (Serves 2)

1 large onion, peeled and quartered
1 large carrot, peeled and cut into 2.5-cm (1-in) chunks
1 medium parsnip, peeled, cut in half and in half again
1 sweet potato or 1 celeriac, peeled and cut into 2.5-cm (1-in) chunks

Cook as for oven-roasted vegetables in Roasted Summer Vegetables recipe (see above).

Stir-fried Vegetables

HED LFD OMSD VEG VG (Serves 2)

Stir-frying is one of the quickest and healthiest ways to cook vegetables. Use whatever vegetables you have available: broccoli, baby
sweetcorn, peppers and mushrooms all work well in stir-fries.

1 dsp sesame oil
1 medium onion, peeled and quartered
1 small carrot, peeled and thinly sliced
6 cauliflower florets
1 medium courgette, thinly sliced
2 tsp grated root ginger
1 tbsp water
1 dsp tamari sauce
salt and black pepper

Heat oil in a deep frying pan or wok. When it begins to sizzle, add
vegetables and ginger. Continue to cook over a high heat for 1
minute, stirring from time to time.

Add 1 tbsp water, turn down heat, cover pan and simmer for a
further 2 minutes or until vegetables are tender, but still crisp. Stir
in tamari sauce, season with salt and black pepper and serve.

Cooking whole grains

Brown rice

Use long-grain rice for savoury dishes and short-grain rice for pud-
dings. Allow ¼ cup uncooked rice per person and three times as
much water as rice. Put rice in a pan with the water and bring to
the boil. Turn down heat, cover pan and simmer for 30–40 minutes
or until all the liquid has been absorbed.

Three ways to spice up rice

Cook rice in vegetable stock and add some frozen peas, chopped
spring onions and sliced mushrooms for the last 10 minutes of
cooking.

Mix in lemon juice, lemon rind and chopped fresh parsley just
before serving.

Add 1 chopped tomato, 1 crushed garlic clove and 1 tsp paprika for
the last 10 minutes of cooking, and mix in chopped fresh coriander
just before serving.

Millet

For 4 people, rinse and drain 1 cup millet. Heat 1 tbsp of olive oil in a heavy-bottomed pan. Add millet to pan and toast it by shaking and stirring until the grains begin to change colour. Add 2 cups boiling stock and 1 tsp salt and bring back to the boil. Turn down heat and cover pan. Cook until all liquid has been absorbed. Remove from heat and let stand for 5 minutes.

Quinoa

For 1 person, use ⅓ cup quinoa. Place in saucepan with 1 cup of boiling water and a little salt. Bring to boil, then turn down heat and simmer, covered, for 10–15 minutes until all the water has been absorbed. When cool, the quinoa can be stored in an airtight container in the fridge for a few days.

Quinoa with Vegetables

HED LFD BBD OMSD VEG VG (Serves 1)

1 small carrot, peeled and thinly sliced
1 small parsnip, peeled and thinly sliced
1 garlic clove, crushed
1 small piece root ginger, peeled and grated
1 dsp olive oil
4 or 5 broccoli florets
½ cup quinoa, cooked as above
1 tbsp extra virgin olive oil
juice of half a lemon
salt and black pepper

Soften carrot, parsnip, garlic and ginger in oil in a covered pan for about 10 minutes. Steam broccoli for 2 minutes in a bowl in the microwave with 1 tbsp of water. When vegetables are cooked, add quinoa and 1 tbsp oil and lemon juice mixed together. Stir well. Season with salt and black pepper.

Salads

The healthiest way to eat vegetables is raw, in salads and salsas. Adding a dressing makes them more interesting and is an easy way of consuming beneficial EFA oils.

Oil and Lemon Dressing

HED LFD OMSD BBD VEG VG (Serves 2)

1 tbsp extra virgin olive oil
1 tbsp lemon juice (or white wine vinegar or apple cider vinegar)
1 garlic clove, peeled and crushed
salt and black pepper

Use Oil and Lemon Dressing on the following salads:

- sliced fennel, grated carrot and chopped dessert apple;
- sliced tomatoes, chopped spring onions and a handful of chopped fresh basil;
- grated carrots, currants, chopped fresh parsley and ½ tsp ground cumin;
- sliced red pepper, celery and sliced cucumber (no need to peel the cucumber).

Green Salad

HED LFD OMSD BBD VEG VG

Use a mixture of salad leaves such as Cos, Little Gem, Webbs Wonderful, Chinese leaves, watercress, salad cress or baby spinach leaves. Tear leaves into small pieces and rinse well in a colander. You can add thinly sliced cucumber as well if desired.

Toss in Oil and Lemon Dressing (see above) just before serving.

Yogurt

Probiotic or 'friendly' bacteria, which are found in live 'bio' yogurt, improve intestinal health, promote good digestion, boost immunity and increase resistance to infection. Probiotics can also help conditions such as IBS and recurrent candida infections. Yogurt is a useful low-fat substitute for cream in dessert recipes and is an ideal basis for flavoured marinades for chicken or fish.

Yogurt Dressing

HED LFD OMSD VEG VG (Serves 2)

2 tbsp yogurt
1 tsp French mustard
salt and black pepper

Use Yogurt Dressing with these salads:

- quartered baby beets, chopped apple, sliced radishes and chopped chives;
- sliced celery, sliced cucumber, chopped apple and chopped walnuts;
- boiled new potatoes and chopped spring onions.

Coleslaw

HED LFD VEG VG (Serves 2)

Mix grated celeriac and carrots with shredded white cabbage and chopped spring onions. Add the juice of half a lemon and 1 crushed garlic clove to the Yogurt Dressing and mix everything together.

Salad Niçoise

HED LFD BBD OMSD (Serves 4)

This family favourite is an example of how a salad can be a main meal. For the OMSD, leave out the eggs.

450 g (1 lb) small new potatoes, scrubbed
2 Little Gem lettuces
4 hard-boiled eggs
2 x 185-g cans tuna chunks, drained
1 can anchovy fillets, drained
4 medium-sized tomatoes, quartered
½ cucumber, thinly sliced
1 small green pepper, deseeded and sliced
12 black olives, pitted

For the dressing
½ cup extra virgin olive oil
juice of 1 lemon
1 large garlic clove, peeled and crushed
1 dsp Dijon mustard
salt and black pepper

Cook potatoes in boiling water for 20 minutes and drain well. Rinse individual lettuce leaves in cold water and shake dry. Shell eggs and slice. Flake tuna and cut anchovies in half. Mix together ingredients for dressing. Put salad ingredients in a large bowl and pour dressing over.

Fish

Buying fish

Fish is such a crucial part of a healthy diet for everyone in the world that it's important, whenever possible, to choose fish from a sustainable source. Some varieties of deep-sea fish, such as cod, have been overfished for generations. Good alternatives to cod are New Zealand hoki, Alaskan pollock, hake and coley. Look out, too, for Alaskan salmon – another sustainable fish.

Buy fish with clear, bright eyes as this indicates freshness. The flesh should be firm and there should be no unpleasant smell. Cutlets and fillets are much easier to cook than whole fish; the fishmonger will gut or fillet the fish for you if necessary.

Canned fish, such as tuna, salmon, sardines and anchovies, are useful standbys for the times when you can't get hold of fresh or frozen fish, but remember that the heat and pressure used in the canning process will reduce the amount of EFAs in the end product.

Cooking fish

Fish is the ultimate fast food. Frying is a traditional way of cooking it, but steaming, poaching, grilling and baking are healthier alternatives and just as quick. My favourite way to cook fish is to brush it with a marinade and then either grill or bake it. If you marinade the fish an hour or so before cooking it, the flavour will be enhanced. Here are two useful marinades – the quantity is enough for two fillets.

Lemon and Ginger Marinade

HED LFD BBD OMSD VEG VG (Serves 2)

juice of half a lemon
1 dsp olive oil
1 garlic clove, peeled and crushed
1 dsp grated fresh ginger root
salt and black pepper

Orange and Tomato Marinade

HED LFD BBD OMSD VEG VG (Serves 2)

1 tbsp orange juice
1 tsp tomato purée
1 garlic clove, peeled and crushed
½ tsp dried thyme
1 dsp olive oil
salt and black pepper

Baked Salmon

HED LFD BBD OMSD WD (Serves 2)

Use two salmon steaks, weighing about 100–115 g (3½–4 oz) each. Heat oven to 180 °C (350 °F, gas mark 4). Place fish steaks on an oiled baking sheet and brush with Lemon and Ginger Marinade (page 112). Cook for 25 minutes, or until fish becomes opaque and flakes when pricked with the point of a knife.

Grilled Salmon

Heat grill. Place fish steaks on an oiled baking sheet and brush with chosen marinade. Cook for about 6 minutes each side.

Grilled Mackerel

HED LFD BBD OMSD WD (Serves 2)

Use 2 medium-sized mackerel fillets weighing about 115 g (4 oz) each Heat grill. Place fillets on an oiled grill pan, skin-side down, and brush with Orange and Tomato Marinade (see above). Cook for about 8 minutes or until fish flakes easily.

Trout can be grilled in the same way as mackerel, using Lemon and Ginger Marinade (page 112).

Courgette and Anchovy Pasta

HED LFD BBD OMSD (Serves 1)

115 g (4 oz) pasta shapes (GF for BBD)
1 medium courgette, halved lengthways and sliced
1 dsp olive oil
2 garlic cloves, crushed
pinch chilli flakes
1 tin anchovies, drained, rinsed and chopped
a few broccoli florets

Start pasta cooking in a pan of boiling water. Soften courgettes in oil in another pan for 5 minutes over a low heat, then add garlic, chilli flakes and anchovies. Cover pan and continue to cook gently. Meanwhile, add broccoli to pasta pan for last 5 minutes. When pasta is cooked, drain and add it and broccoli to courgette and anchovy mixture.

Sardine Pasta

HED LFD BBD OMSD (Serves 1)

1 celery stick, sliced
1 garlic clove, crushed
½ red pepper, deseeded and sliced
½ small courgette, sliced
1 dsp olive oil
200 ml (7 fl oz) passata
1 tin sardines, drained and chopped
1 tsp paprika
1 tsp dried parsley
salt

Soften celery, garlic, pepper and courgette in oil in a covered pan over a low heat for about 10 minutes. Add passata, sardines, paprika and parsley. Mix well and heat through. Season with salt and serve with your pasta of choice.

Moroccan Baked Fish

HED LFD BBD OMSD WD (Serves 2)

grated rind and juice of half a lemon
1 dsp olive oil
1 tsp harissa powder
salt and black pepper
2 large white fish fillets
10 cherry tomatoes, halved
6 olives, stoned and halved

Preheat oven to 190 °C (375 °F, gas mark 5). Cut a piece of tin foil large enough to wrap around both fish to form a parcel. Mix lemon juice and rind, oil, harissa and a little salt and pepper together in a bowl. Place fish fillets on tin foil, pour over marinade and scatter tomatoes and olives on top. Seal up parcel and bake in the pre-heated oven for 20 minutes.

Using the method described above, you can vary the taste by using different combinations of vegetables and flavourings. For example, sliced leek, tomatoes and lemon with lemon juice and fresh coriander or sliced fennel with lime juice and fresh parsley.

Provençal Fish

HED LFD BBD OMSD WD (Serves 2)

1 dsp olive oil
4 spring onions, chopped
½ green pepper and ½ red pepper, finely chopped
1 x 220-g tin chopped tomatoes
1 dsp flour
pinch chilli flakes
1 tsp Italian herbs seasoning
salt and black pepper
2 white fish fillets

Heat oil in a pan and soften spring onions and peppers for about 5 minutes. Add tomatoes, flour, chilli and herbs and season with salt and black pepper. Mix everything together well. Add fish fillets to mixture, cover pan and simmer for 10 minutes.

Poultry and meat dishes

Healthier ways to eat meat

Buy good-quality poultry and meat from a reputable supplier. Choose lean cuts of meat with as little visible fat as possible.

Chicken and turkey breasts are leaner without the skin. Leg of lamb is less fatty than beef or pork, while offal (liver and kidneys), in addition to being relatively low in saturated fat, contains beneficial complex fatty acids.

When grilling or roasting poultry or meat, place them on a rack in a roasting dish to drain away excess fat. This is especially important if you are cooking high-fat convenience foods such as sausages or burgers.

An average adult portion of poultry or meat is 115 g (4 oz). When cooking meat, look for recipes that combine meat with lentils or beans (such as Chilli con Carne, page 120) as then you will need less meat per person. This makes for a lower-fat meal, but tastes good enough for you not to miss the extra poultry or meat.

Liver and kidneys can be cooked in casseroles or sauces instead of frying them (such as Liver and Onion Casserole, page 122).

Note that those on the low-fat diet should eat no red meat in the first year of the diet, but may start eating one red meat dish per week in the second year.

Those on the Best Bet diet may eat one red meat dish per week, if desired.

Paprika Chicken

HED LFD BBD WD (Serves 2)

225 g (8 oz) chicken breast, cut into 6 pieces

For the marinade
1 tbsp olive oil
1 garlic clove, crushed, or 1 tsp garlic purée
2 tsp paprika
1 tsp ground cumin
¼ tsp salt

Mix together the marinade ingredients in a large bowl. Add chicken pieces to bowl and coat well with marinade, then leave to marinate for at least an hour in a cool place or the fridge.

Lay chicken pieces on a baking sheet and grill for 10 minutes. Turn over and cook other side for 5 or 6 minutes until cooked through.

Here are two alternative marinades for chicken.

Lemon Herb Marinade

HED LFD BBD OMSD VEG VG (Serves 2)

1 dsp olive oil
juice of half a lemon
1 garlic clove, crushed, or 1 tsp garlic purée
1 tsp Italian herb seasoning or dried parsley
¼ tsp salt

Spicy Middle Eastern Marinade

HED LFD BBD OMSD VEG VG (Serves 2)

1 tbsp olive oil
2 tsp harissa powder
1 tsp ground cumin
1 tsp garlic purée
pinch of salt

Roast Chicken and Vegetables

HED LFD BBD WD (Serves 2)

Coat chicken pieces in Lemon Herb Marinade (see above) and cook with Roasted Summer Vegetables (page 106).

Jambalaya

HED LFD BBD WD (Serves 4)

This is a low-fat version of a Creole dish and makes a great family meal for special occasions.

175 g (6 oz) long-grain brown rice
900 ml (1½ pt) chicken stock
1 tbsp olive oil
450 g (1 lb) chicken breasts, cubed
4 celery sticks, sliced
2 green peppers, deseeded and sliced
4 large tomatoes, chopped
2 garlic cloves, crushed
3 tsp paprika
¼ tsp cayenne pepper
1 tsp dried oregano
1 bay leaf
1 x 250-g (9-oz) packet cooked frozen jumbo prawns, defrosted
6 spring onions, chopped
salt and black pepper

Cook rice in chicken stock in a covered pan for about 35 minutes. In a large pan, brown chicken pieces all over in oil, then remove from pan and set aside. Add celery and peppers to pan and cook gently for 10 minutes until soft. Add tomatoes, garlic, spices and herbs and leave to simmer, covered, for a further 10 minutes. Add cooked rice to chicken and vegetables, together with prawns and spring onions, and mix well. Heat through for about 5 minutes, adding a little hot water if necessary to prevent sticking. Season with salt and black pepper.

Oriental Chicken

HED LFD (Serves 2)

300 ml (½ pt) vegetable stock
1 x 2.5-cm (1-in) piece ginger root, peeled and grated
1 garlic clove, sliced
1 tbsp tamari sauce
1 carrot, sliced very thinly
2 small chicken breasts (about 230 g (8 oz) in total), cut into strips
60 g (2 oz) mushrooms, sliced
1 small courgette, thinly sliced
½ bunch spring onions, chopped
1 dsp cornflour mixed with 1 dsp water
black pepper

Simmer the first 6 ingredients together for 5 minutes in a pan. Add mushrooms and courgette and simmer for a further 5 minutes. Add spring onions and cornflour mixture and cook for 1 minute more. Season with black pepper before serving.

Chicken Korma

HED LFD BBD (Serves 2)

I don't usually advocate using ready-made sauces or pastes, but Geo curry pastes, which are available from retailers such as Healthy Supplies, are made from organic natural ingredients and are dairy- and wheat-free (see Useful addresses).

2 chicken breasts, cut into bite-sized pieces
1 tbsp olive oil
2 tbsp Geo korma curry paste
1 large carrot, peeled and either grated or chopped
2 tomatoes, chopped
1 dsp rice flour
150 ml (¼ pt) hot water
½ tsp salt

Brown chicken pieces in oil in a frying pan. Add curry paste and mix well with chicken. Add remaining ingredients, bring to boil, turn down heat and simmer, covered, for 15 minutes.

Chicken Kebabs

HED LFD BBD WD (Serves 2)

Cut chicken breast into 2.5-cm (1-in) cubes and marinate in Spicy Middle Eastern Marinade (page 117). Thread the chicken pieces on to 2 skewers, interspersed with cherry tomatoes, whole button mushrooms and thick slices of courgette. Either grill or barbecue, turning at regular intervals to cook thoroughly.

Chilli con Carne

HED (Serves 4)

This recipe also works well with minced chicken or turkey instead of beef. Serve with rice or in a wholemeal wrap or tortilla with shredded lettuce and cucumber.

1 medium onion, peeled and sliced
1 dsp olive oil
2 garlic cloves, peeled and crushed
175 g (12 oz) lean beef mince
2 heaped dsp flour
2 x 400-g (14-oz) can chopped tomatoes
1 x 400-g (14-oz) can kidney beans, drained and rinsed
1 green pepper, deseeded and chopped
½ tsp chilli powder
1 tsp paprika

In a large pan, soften onion in olive oil over a low heat for 10 minutes.

Stir in garlic and cook another minute. Now push onions to side of pan and add mince. Raise heat and quickly brown meat, stirring to get rid of lumps.

Stir in flour, then remaining ingredients. Bring mixture to boil, then turn down heat, cover and simmer for 30 minutes.

Barbecued Lamb Kebabs

HED (Serves 4)

450 g (1 lb) lean lamb, cubed
a few cherry tomatoes
1 courgette, sliced
a few button mushrooms

Marinade
2 tbsp olive oil
2 tsp runny honey
2 tsp French mustard
1 tbsp tomato purée
1 tsp mixed dried herbs
½ tsp salt

Make marinade with oil, honey, mustard, tomato purée, herbs and salt and put in a large bowl. Add meat to bowl and mix well so meat is coated in marinade and leave to marinate for at least an hour in a cool place or fridge. Thread marinated meat on to skewers, interspersed with cherry tomatoes, courgette slices and button mushrooms. Cook under grill or on a barbecue, turning from time to time to cook thoroughly.

Pork with Apples

HED (Serves 4)

1 onion, sliced
1 tbsp olive oil
450 g (1 lb) lean pork, cubed
3 dsp flour
2 medium carrots, peeled and sliced
2 eating apples, peeled, cored and sliced
600 ml (1 pt) chicken stock
1 dsp Dijon mustard
handful fresh sage leaves, chopped

Soften onion in oil in a large pan for 5 minutes. Add pork to pan and brown pieces all over. Add flour and mix well. Add carrots, apples, chicken stock and mustard and bring to boil. Turn down heat, cover and simmer gently for about 45 minutes. Add sage leaves for final 5 minutes.

Liver and Onion Casserole

HED LFD WD (Serves 2)

1 large onion, sliced
1 tbsp olive oil
175 g (6 oz) lamb's liver, sliced thinly
1 cup sliced button mushrooms
180 ml (6 fl oz) vegetable stock
1 dsp French mustard
1 dsp corn or maize flour dissolved in 1 tbsp water

Preheat oven to 190 °C (375 °F, gas mark 5). Soften onion in oil in a large frying pan over a low heat for 5 minutes.

Push onion to sides of pan and add liver slices. Add another dsp oil if necessary and brown liver on both sides. Remove onion and liver and place in a casserole dish with mushrooms.

Put stock, mustard and cornflour mixture in pan and heat, stirring, until sauce has thickened. Pour into casserole over onion and liver, cover and cook for 25 minutes in the preheated oven.

Vegetarian dishes

Egg and Cashew Nut Pilau

HED LFD BBD OMSD VEG (Serves 2)

For a change, replace the nuts with 55 g (2 oz) sliced mushrooms. For the OMSD, leave out the eggs.

½ cup of brown rice
½ tsp ground turmeric
½ bunch spring onions, chopped
1 garlic clove, crushed, or 1 tsp garlic purée
1 tsp olive oil
2 tsp mild curry powder
1 tsp garam masala
1 tsp ground cumin
1 small green pepper, deseeded and sliced
¼ cup raisins
¼ cup cashew nuts
2 hard-boiled eggs, sliced
salt and black pepper

Cook rice with turmeric in 1½ cups water for 30 minutes. Drain well.

Meanwhile, cook spring onions and garlic gently in oil in a large frying pan for 5 minutes. Mix in spices and cook for another minute. Add green pepper, raisins and nuts and continue to cook over a low heat, stirring from time to time, for a further 5 minutes. Add a little water if necessary to prevent sticking.

Shell and slice the hard-boiled eggs and add to pan. Last, add the rice and mix everything together well. Season to taste with salt and black pepper.

Turmeric

Turmeric has a very long history of being used medicinally and has been the subject of over 5,000 biomedical studies. The active ingredient is curcumin, which gives it its vivid yellow colour. It is antiviral, antifungal, antibacterial and anti-inflammatory. It contains antioxidants, which help to fight free radicals, and its neuroprotective actions support better memory and cognitive function. To gain the maximum benefit from turmeric, take it with a fatty liquid, such as coconut milk, or add to a recipe that contains olive oil.

Stuffed Aubergine

HED LFD BBD OMSD VEG VG (Serves 2)

1 large aubergine
little olive oil
1 celery stick, sliced
2 large garlic cloves, crushed
2 large tomatoes, chopped
1 tsp ground cumin
¼ tsp chilli powder
25 g black olives, pitted and halved
fresh parsley, basil or coriander
salt and black pepper

To serve
little low-fat cheese, grated (HED, LFD, VEG), or handful of pine nuts, toasted (BBD, OMSD, VG)

Preheat oven to 200 °C (400 °F, gas mark 6). Slice aubergine in half. Scrape out flesh to within 1 cm (½ in) of skin and reserve. Brush shells with olive oil and place in baking dish. Cover with foil and bake in the preheated oven for 20 minutes.

Soften celery, garlic and reserved scraped-out aubergine flesh in olive oil in covered pan. Add tomatoes and spices and cook for 3 minutes. Stir in olives and herbs and season well with salt and black pepper. Pile this stuffing into baked aubergine shells and sprinkle with either low-fat grated cheese or toasted pine nuts. Reduce oven temperature to 180 °C (350 °F, gas mark 4) and bake for 20 minutes.

Here is an alternative stuffing mix.

scraped-out flesh from aubergine, as before
1 small onion, chopped
1 garlic clove, crushed
2 tomatoes, chopped
225 g (4 oz) chopped nuts
30 g (1 oz) sultanas
1 tbsp fresh parsley, chopped
1 tsp each ground cumin, coriander and garam masala

Black Bean and Kidney Bean Chilli

HED LFD OMSD VEG VG (Serves 4)

2 large carrots, grated or chopped finely
2 garlic cloves, crushed
1 x 400-g (14-oz) tin passata plus ½ tin of water
1 x 400-g (14-oz) tin black beans, drained and rinsed
1 x 400-g (14-oz) tin kidney beans, drained and rinsed
1 green pepper, deseeded and chopped
1 tsp chilli flakes
salt and black pepper

To serve
4 portions cooked rice or quinoa

Place all ingredients in a large pan and simmer for about 10 minutes until they are heated through and carrots are soft. Serve with rice or quinoa.

Lentil and Pea Dahl

HED LFD OMSD VEG VG (Serves 2)

375 ml (12½ fl oz) water
125 g (4 oz) dried red lentils, rinsed
1 dsp olive oil
2 celery sticks, sliced
2 garlic cloves, crushed
1 tsp ground ginger
½ tsp chilli powder
1 tsp turmeric
1 tsp ground coriander
100 ml (3 fl oz) water
1 dsp tomato purée
75 g (2½ oz) cooked peas
salt

To serve
2 portions cooked rice or quinoa

Bring water to boil and add rinsed lentils. Cover and simmer for 10 minutes or until liquid has been absorbed.

Heat oil in pan and soften celery and garlic. Add spices, water and tomato purée and cook for 10 minutes. Combine lentils with celery and garlic sauce and add peas. Season with salt and serve with rice or quinoa.

Fruity desserts

Apple Snow

HED LFD BBD OMSD VEG VG (Serves 1)

Simmer a sliced cooking apple with 1 dsp honey and 2 tbsp water over a low heat until mushy. Put apples in a heatproof bowl, cover with two stiffly beaten egg whites and brown under the grill. An alternative to apples would be apricots or rhubarb.

Fruit Fool

HED LFD OMSD WD VEG VG (Serves 1)

Mix summer berries such as raspberries, strawberries or blackberries with a little runny honey and a cup of yogurt (OMSD and VG, use soya yogurt; WD, use coconut yogurt). Blend in food processor.

Baked Banana

HED LFD BBD OMSD VEG VG (Serves 1)

Peel a banana and slice lengthwise. Place in a heatproof bowl, pour over the juice of 1 orange and scatter with crushed hazelnuts. Cook on high in the microwave for 1¼ minutes.

Baked Apples

HED LFD BBD OMSD VEG VG (Serves 2)

2 dessert apples
2 dsp raisins
1 tsp ground cinnamon
1 tbsp runny honey
3 tbsp water

Preheat oven to 200 °C (400 °F, gas mark 6). Core apples and place in a baking dish. Stuff centre with raisins and sprinkle cinnamon and honey over each hole. Add water to baking dish and bake for 30 minutes.

Fruit Salad

HED LFD BBD OMSD VEG VG

Put a mixture of fruit, such as sliced banana, kiwi fruit, apple or pear, in a bowl with some seedless grapes or fresh strawberries. Cover with fruit juice, such as orange or apple and mango. You can add some tinned fruit, such as pineapple, or mix fresh fruit with dried fruit.

Apricot and Banana Granola Crumble in the Microwave

HED LFD BBD VEG VG (Serves 4)

125 g (4 oz) dried apricots
1 cup water
2 large bananas, sliced

For the crumble topping
90 g (3 oz) flour
½ tsp ground cinnamon
60 g (2 oz) Pure sunflower margarine
30 g (1 oz) nuts, chopped
60 g (2 oz) granola or rice flakes
30 g (1 oz) muscovado sugar

Place apricots and water in a 230-mm (8-in) diameter glass casserole dish and heat in microwave on high for 3 minutes. Mix sliced bananas with apricots.

For the crumble topping, mix flour with cinnamon and rub in margarine until the mixture resembles fine breadcrumbs. Mix in nuts, granola or rice flakes and sugar. Use mixture to cover fruit in bowl. Cook on high for 6–7 minutes.

Cinnamon

The spice cinnamon, used in cooking and baking since medieval times, contains large amounts of antioxidants, some of which are anti-inflammatory. It also has antifungal and antibacterial properties. Scientific studies have also suggested that it may have beneficial effects on neurodegenerative disease. In larger doses, it lowers blood sugar levels and has a powerful antidiabetic effect.

There are two types of cinnamon: Cassia and Ceylon. If you want to benefit from its therapeutic properties, Ceylon cinnamon (found in health food shops) is preferable. Use it in porridge or smoothies or add to herb teas.

Cashew Nut Cream

HED LFD BBD OMSD VEG VG (Serves 2)

This is a dairy-free alternative to cow's milk or yogurt to serve with your fruity desserts.

1 cup raw cashew nuts, soaked for 4 hours
½ cup water
1 dsp maple syrup or honey
½ tsp vanilla extract
pinch sea salt

Drain nuts, then put in food processor with all the other ingredients and blend on high until thick and creamy. This may take some time. If it's too thick, add a little more water and blend again.

Baking

Healthy treats

Everyone likes to indulge in sweet treats from time to time, but is it possible to bake a 'healthy' cake? Yes, I think it is. Here are some guidelines.

- Replace standard white flour with either a good-quality unbleached white flour, such as Doves Farm, or well-sieved wholemeal flour.
- Replace white sugar with dried fruit, fruit purée or honey.
- Fat should be kept to a minimum and taken in the form of unrefined oils or unhydrogenated margarine (such as Pure). Replace 1 egg with 2 fat-free egg whites.
- The addition of nuts makes cakes even more nutritious and grated carrot gives a lovely moist texture.

Here's an example of healthy baking that even people with a sweet tooth like.

Honey Oat Bars

HED VEG VG

1 cup rolled oats
1 cup sultanas
¼ cup chopped dried apricots
½ cup self-raising flour
½ cup coconut flakes
⅓ cup unhydrogenated margarine
¼ cup honey

Preheat oven to 190 °C (375 °F, gas mark 5). Mix together oats, sultanas, apricots, flour and coconut flakes.

Melt margarine and honey in a glass bowl or microwave saucepan in a microwave and mix in the other ingredients.

Grease a 175-mm (7-in) diameter sponge cake tin and pour mixture in. Bake in the preheated oven for 20 minutes. Cut into wedges while still warm and in the tin. (Don't worry if it seems soft – it will harden up as it cools.) Leave to cool before removing from the tin.

Gluten-free baking

Cooking with gluten-free (GF) flour requires a different technique from those used in conventional baking. This is because gluten is the binding agent in the grain; it helps the crumbs to stick together and makes dough elastic enough to knead. Here are some tips for making gluten-free bread, cakes or pastry.

As a general rule . . .

For best results, use a mixture of different GF flours, such as a blend of 3 parts brown rice flour, 2 parts tapioca flour and 1 part maize flour.

You can compensate for the lack of gluten by adding one of the following:

- 1 tsp xanthan gum to every 170 g (6 oz) plain GF flour;
- 1 part Orgran No Gluten to 5 parts plain GF flour.

Some GF flours deteriorate quickly so, once opened, store your packets of GF flour in plastic containers in the freezer. They won't solidify and will keep for up to three months.

Bread and cakes

Soda bread (bread made without yeast) and cakes made without sugar will not stay fresh as long as their conventional counterparts. Soda bread may be cut up into individual portions and stored in sandwich bags in the freezer until required. Cakes and muffins will keep up to five days in a plastic box in the fridge or up to a month in the freezer.

GF bread and cakes taste better if they have been 'refreshed' in the microwave before eating. Heat two muffins or two slices of bread on medium high for 1 minute or, if frozen, on defrost for 2 minutes.

Pastry

To 'rub in', lightly use your fingertips to rub the margarine into the flour, lifting the mixture as you do so, until it resembles breadcrumbs.

To make pastry dough, add the exact amount of cold water speci-fied and bring water and crumbs together with a palette knife. Use your well-floured hands to finish forming the dough ball. Add a little extra water if it's too dry or a bit more flour if it's too sticky.

Chill the pastry in the fridge for 30 minutes before rolling out. Dough can be wrapped in cling film and kept in the fridge for two to three days before use.

Lifting up a large sheet of GF pastry without it breaking is a near impossibility as it is very fragile. Small individual pies are fine as the circle of pastry is small enough to be picked up on a large spatula. Turn large pies into a 'cobbler', forming the crust by overlapping small circles of pastry. You can use an upturned tumbler to cut these out.

Gluten-free Soda Bread

HED LFD BBD OMSD V

If you can't find millet flour, use millet flakes and blitz in a food processor to form flour.

300 ml (½ pt) milk
1 tsp vinegar
1¾ cups plain GF flour
⅔ cup millet flour
¼ cup Orgran No Gluten
2 tsp baking soda
1 tsp salt

Preheat oven to 200 °C (400 °F, gas mark 6). Grease a baking sheet. Mix milk and vinegar and leave for 10 minutes. Mix all dry ingre-dients together in a bowl, then add the milk and vinegar mixture. Mix with a metal spoon to form a ball of dough. If the mixture is too dry, add more water a little at a time. Flour your hands and roll the ball on to the greased baking sheet. Flatten slightly and form a cross on the top with a knife. Bake in the preheated oven for 30 minutes, until a knife inserted into the centre comes out dry. Leave to cool for 30 minutes before slicing.

Corn Bread

HED LFD BBD OMSD VEG VG

1⅔ cups maize flour or polenta
⅔ cup brown rice flour
2 tsp baking powder
1 tsp salt
1 tsp chilli flakes
2 tsp xanthan gum
1 small red pepper, finely diced
1 cup milk
½ cup water
3 tbsp olive oil

Preheat oven to 200 °C (400 °F, gas mark 6). Grease and flour a 450-g (1-lb) loaf tin.

Mix dry ingredients together in a bowl and add diced red pepper. Whisk liquid ingredients together and add to bowl with dry ingredients. Mix well. Put mixture in the prepared loaf tin and bake in the preheated oven for 30 minutes. Leave to cool for 30 minutes before cutting.

Apricot Tea Bread

HED LFD OMSD VEG VG

1 x 400-g (14-oz) tin apricots in fruit juice
300 ml (10 oz) plain yogurt (OMSD and VG, use soya yogurt)
250 g (9 oz) brown rice flour
1 tsp ground cinnamon
1 tsp allspice
1 tsp ground nutmeg
2 tsp baking powder
140 g (5 oz) currants or raisins

Preheat oven to 180 °C (350 °F, gas mark 4). Grease and flour a 450-g (1lb) loaf tin.

Empty apricots and fruit juice into food processor and whizz to a purée. Add yogurt, flour, spices and baking powder and mix well.

Mix in currants or raisins by hand, then pour mixture into prepared loaf tin. Bake in the preheated oven for 40–45 minutes, until a skewer inserted into the centre comes out clean. Leave to cool for 30 minutes before turning out.

Peach Muffins

HED LFD BBD OMSD VEG VG (Makes 6 large or 9 smaller muffins)

This simple method for making muffins uses canned fruit to provide flavour and sweetness, so you don't need to add either sugar or eggs. I find them quite sweet enough as they are, but you can add a dessertspoon of honey to the recipe if you prefer. For best results, heat gently in a microwave before eating.

1 x 400-g (14-oz) can peaches in juice
1½ cups Orgran self-raising GF flour
3 level tbsp unhydrogenated dairy-free margarine, such as Pure
1 tsp vanilla extract
½ cup sultanas

Preheat oven to 200 °C (400 °F, gas mark 6). Lightly grease a muffin tray.

Make a purée of peaches and their juice in a food processor.

Add flour, margarine and vanilla extract and blend again. Mix in sultanas by hand. Spoon mixture into prepared muffin tray and bake in the preheated oven for 25 minutes, Leave to cool for 10 minutes before removing muffins from the tray.

Pear and Carob Muffins

HED LFD OMSD VEG VG (Makes 6 large or 9 smaller muffins)

Replace peaches with a can of pears in juice and add 2 dsp of carob powder.

Apricot Muffins

HED LFD OMSD VEG VG (Makes 6 large or 9 smaller muffins)

Replace peaches with a can of apricots in juice and add 1 tsp ground cinnamon to mix.

Recipes for the Wahls diet

Because the Wahls diet is quite different from the other diets in this book in its use of fats and protein, I recommend that you check out the recipe section in *The Wahls Protocol* for examples of typical recipes and menu plans. However, here are some recipes inspired by those in the book to get you started.

Wahls Green Smoothie

(Serves 1)

2 celery sticks
1 kiwi fruit, peeled
1 pear, peeled and cored
1 x 7-cm (3-in) section of unpeeled cucumber
4 broccoli florets or handful of fresh spinach leaves
½ cup coconut or almond milk

Whizz all the ingredients together in a food processor or blender.

Bone Broth

1 large onion, unpeeled and chopped
3 garlic cloves
1 tsp kelp powder or 1 tbsp dulce flakes
2 tsp sea salt
carcase of a 2.25-kg (5-lb) chicken
vegetables, such as 1 large carrot and 2 large celery sticks, sliced
4 tbsp organic apple cider vinegar
4.5 litres (8 pints) of water

Place all the ingredients in a large pot and bring to the boil. Turn down heat and simmer, covered, for 2 hours. Skim off any foam, then drain broth into another pan and stand pan in cold water in sink to cool it down rapidly. The broth can then be stored in a sealed container in the fridge for up to 3 days or in a freezer for 3 months.

Chicken Livers with Bacon

(Serves 4)

230 g (8 oz) lean bacon, chopped into pieces
230 g (8 oz) mushrooms, sliced
1 tsp kelp powder
2 onions, peeled and sliced
450 g (1 lb) chicken livers, gristle removed, chopped
1 tbsp apple cider vinegar
½ tsp sea salt

Fry bacon in a frying pan until it begins to brown in places. Pour off excess fat. Add mushrooms, kelp powder and onions and cook over a medium heat for 5 minutes. Stir in chicken livers, cider vinegar and salt and cook for another 3 minutes.

Algerian Chicken

(Serves 4)

1 tbsp coconut oil
680 g (1½ lbs) chicken pieces (breast, legs or thighs)
4 garlic cloves, crushed
2 tsp turmeric
1 tsp cinnamon
1 x 400-g (14-oz) can chopped tomatoes
2 cups sliced leeks
1 cup Bone Broth (page 135)
1 red pepper, deseeded and sliced
1 medium carrot, sliced
1 tsp kelp powder
½ tsp salt
4 cups green beans or asparagus
2 cups chopped broccoli

Heat coconut oil in a large pan and brown chicken pieces all over. Add garlic and spices and mix well. Then add everything else except the green vegetables and simmer for 15 minutes over medium heat. Add the green vegetables and simmer for another 5 minutes mutil tender.

Sample menus

These menus are examples of what you could eat on each of the first four featured diets, but bear in mind the following points.

- You may need to adapt the menus to accommodate individual food intolerances.
- The menus assume you are snacking on fruit and vegetables to make up your five a day.
- Vegetarian dishes are included in all the menus as they are naturally low in fat and have a high vegetable content.
- Use whatever fruit and vegetables are in season (see Table 3.1, page 34).
- If you are on the low-fat diet, you may add one portion of red meat per week after the first year. On the Best Bet diet, you may also eat one portion of red meat a week if you wish. In each case, make sure the remaining meals you eat that day are low in saturated fat.

If you wish to follow the Wahls diet, I suggest you refer to the very detailed weekly menu plan in *The Wahls Protocol*.

The healthy eating diet

Monday

Breakfast: Low-sugar muesli with skimmed milk and sliced banana

Lunch: Ham and salad sandwich in wholemeal bread; orange

Dinner: Moroccan Baked Fish (page 115) with new potatoes and steamed broccoli;

Marinated Spiced Fruit (page 94) with natural yogurt

Tuesday

Breakfast: Small glass fruit juice; boiled egg and two slices of wholemeal toast with low-fat spread

Lunch: Baked potato (page 102) with tuna and low-fat mayonnaise and Green Salad (page 109); apple

Dinner: Chilli con Carne (page 120) with rice (page 107) and sweetcorn; half a small melon

Wednesday

Breakfast: Porridge (page 92) with skimmed milk and a banana

Lunch: Middle Eastern Lentil Soup (page 95) with a wholemeal roll and low-fat spread; Peach Muffin (page 134)

Dinner: Paprika Chicken (page 117), brown rice (page 107) with peas, mushrooms and spinach; plain yogurt with mixed berries and a drizzle of honey

Thursday

Breakfast: Fruit Smoothie (page 94); grilled bacon, tomatoes and mushrooms

Lunch: Salmon and cucumber sandwich in wholemeal bread; pear

Dinner: Lean lamb chop with Indian Spiced Wedges (page 103) and steamed cabbage; Apple Snow (page 127)

Friday

Breakfast: Half a grapefruit; small tin reduced-sugar baked beans on wholemeal toast

Lunch: Broccoli and Courgette Soup (page 97) and wholegrain cracker (such as Ryvita) with sliced ham; Pear and Carob Muffin (page 134)

Dinner: Sardine Pasta (page 114); Granola (page 93) with skimmed milk and chopped apple

Saturday

Breakfast: Marinated Spiced Fruit (page 94) with plain yogurt; wholemeal toast and honey

Lunch: Baked potato (page 102) with grated half-fat Cheddar cheese and Green Salad (page 109); peach or nectarine

Dinner: Grilled Mackerel with Sweet Potato Wedges (pages 113 and 103), cauliflower and peas; Fruit Fool (page 127)

Sunday

Breakfast: Half a small melon; wholegrain cereal with skimmed milk and sultanas

Lunch: Mushroom omelette with tomato salad and cress; Honey Oat Bar (page 130)

Dinner: Roast Chicken and Vegetables (page 117) and brown rice (page 107); Apricot and Banana Granola Crumble (page 128)

Snacks

● Packets of peanuts and raisins.
● Mix of almonds and dried apricots.
● Wholegrain crackers (such as Ryvita), rice cakes or oatcakes with cottage cheese or a dip, such as Hummus or Sardine Pâté (pages 100 and 101).
● Fresh fruit, dried fruit, fruit smoothies.
● Fruit muffins or Honey Oat Bars (pages 134 and 130).

Low-fat diet

Monday

Breakfast: Marinated Spiced Fruit (page 94); Porridge (page 92) with skimmed milk and teaspoon of honey

Lunch: Baked potato (page 102) with chopped chicken, Yogurt Dressing (page 110) with fresh coriander on a mixed salad; apple

Dinner: Black Bean and Kidney Bean Chilli (page 125) with brown rice (page 107) and steamed kale; Peach Muffin (page 134)

Tuesday

Breakfast: Small glass fruit juice; wholegrain cereal with skimmed milk and sultanas

Lunch: Sweet Potato and Coriander Soup (page 96); wholemeal toast with Salmon Pâté (page 100); pear

Dinner: Oriental Chicken with lemon rice and Green Salad (pages 119, 107 and 109); Granola Delight (page 94)

Wednesday

Breakfast: Half a grapefruit; small tin low-sugar baked beans on wholemeal toast

Lunch: Quinoa (page 108) with vegetables and sliced turkey; fruit salad with plain yogurt

Dinner: Oven-roasted Vegetables with Pasta and Cashew Nuts (page 106); Apple Snow (page 127)

Thursday

Breakfast: Granola (page 93) with skimmed milk and berries; wholegrain cracker (such as Ryvita) with reduced-sugar jam

Lunch: Low-fat or home-made Hummus (page 100) with wholemeal toast and vegetable sticks; banana

Dinner: Baked Salmon (page 113) with new potatoes, steamed broccoli and carrots; Pear and Carob Muffin (page 134)

Friday

Breakfast: Half a small melon; boiled egg with wholemeal toast and a low-fat spread

Lunch: Minestrone Soup with Corn Bread (pages 99 and 133); apple

Dinner: Courgette and Anchovy Pasta (page 114) with tomato and basil salad; Marinated Spiced Fruit (page 94) and plain yogurt

Saturday

Breakfast: Reduced-sugar muesli with skimmed milk and fresh berries

Lunch: Fresh olives; turkey and salad sandwich made with wholemeal bread

Dinner: Provençal Fish with Potato Wedges (pages 115 and 103) and spinach; Baked Banana (page 127)

Sunday

Breakfast: Fruit Smoothie (page 94); wholemeal toast with tahini and sliced tomato

Lunch: Baked potato (page 102) with cottage cheese and chives and a fennel salad; orange

Dinner: Chicken Korma (page 119) with brown rice (page 107 34 0) and steamed green beans; Apricot and Banana Granola Crumble (page 128)

Snacks

- Fruit and nut mix made of raisins, sunflower seeds, pumpkin seeds, cashew nuts and almonds.

- Raw vegetables, such as carrot sticks, celery sticks, cucumber slices, cherry tomatoes, cauliflower florets, olives. Can be eaten alone or with a dip, such as Hummus or Sardine Pâté (pages 100 and 101).
- Rice cakes or wholegrain crackers (such as Ryvita) with tahini.
- Fresh fruit, dried fruit, fruit smoothies.

Best Bet diet

Monday

Breakfast: Porridge (page 92) with rice milk and sliced banana; crispbread with tahini

Lunch: Fish Soup with Corn Bread (pages 98 and 133); apple or pear

Dinner: Grilled Mackerel with Potato Wedges (pages 113 and 103), spring greens and carrots; Peach Muffin (page 134)

Tuesday

Breakfast: Marinated Spiced Fruit (page 94); cooked chicken with sliced avocado

Lunch: Baked potato (page 102) with tuna and passata and Green Salad (page 109); cherries or grapes

Dinner: Egg and Mushroom Pilau (page 123) with spinach; mixed berry fruit salad

Wednesday

Breakfast: Sardines on toasted Gluten-free Soda Bread (page 132) with grilled tomatoes and mushrooms

Lunch: Sweet Potato and Coriander Soup (page 96) and toasted GF bread with tahini; orange

Dinner: Stuffed Aubergine (page 124) with pine nuts, lemon rice (page 107) and Green Salad (page 109); pear

Thursday

Breakfast: Granola (page 93) with rice milk and sliced peach or nectarine; GF toast with nut butter

Lunch: Broccoli and Courgette Soup with Corn Bread (pages 97 and 133) and cold cooked chicken; Apricot Muffin (page 134)

Dinner: Sardine Pasta (page 114) with steamed kale; Apple Snow (page 127)

Friday

Breakfast: Green Smoothie (page 94); toasted Gluten-free Soda Bread (page 132) with nut butter

Lunch: Cock-a-leekie Soup (page 97) and rice cakes with tahini; Coleslaw with Oil and Lemon Dressing (pages 110 and 109)

Dinner: Provençal Fish with Sweet Potato Wedges (pages 115 and 103) and spinach; Baked Banana (page 127)

Saturday

Breakfast: Small glass fruit juice; Porridge (page 92) with rice milk, hazelnuts and chia seeds

Lunch: Baked potato (page 102) with chopped turkey and coriander in Oil and Lemon Dressing (page 109), plus a tomato, cress and celery salad; pear

Dinner: Baked Salmon (page 113) with Stir-fried Vegetables and millet (pages 107 and 108); Marinated Spiced Fruit (page 94)

Sunday

Breakfast: Fruit Smoothie (page 94); toasted Gluten-free Soda Bread and Guacamole (pages 132 and 101)

Lunch: Courgette and Anchovy Pasta (page 114); grapes

Dinner: Jambalaya (page 118) with steamed kale; Apricot and Banana Granola Crumble (page 128)

Snacks

- Fruit and nut mix made of raisins, sunflower seeds, pumpkin seeds, cashew nuts and almonds.
- Raw vegetables, such as carrot sticks, celery sticks, cucumber slices, cherry tomatoes, cauliflower florets, olives. Can be eaten alone or with a dip or Sardine Pâté (page 100).
- Rice cakes or GF crispbread with tahini.
- Fresh fruit, dried fruit, smoothies, GF muffins.

The Overcoming MS diet

Note that 'milk' means soya, nut, rice or oat milk. 'Crispbread' means wholemeal fat-free crispbreads, such as Amisa buckwheat or Ryvita. 'Wholemeal bread' means bread made using unrefined flour and that contains no processed oils or trans fats.

Monday

Breakfast: Granola Delight (page 94) made with fresh berries and soya yogurt; wholemeal toast with Marmite or tahini

Lunch: Middle Eastern Lentil Soup (page 95) with crispbread and Sardine Pâté (page 101); Peach Muffin (page 134)

Dinner: Egg and Mushroom Pilau and Green Salad with Oil and Lemon Dressing (pages 123 and 109); Baked Apple (page 127)

Tuesday

Breakfast: Half a small melon; Porridge (page 92) with banana and milk

Lunch: Baked potato (page 102) with tinned tuna and home-made Coleslaw (page 110); peach or nectarine

Dinner: Black Bean and Kidney Bean Chilli (page 125) with rice (page 107) and steamed kale; Marinated Spiced Fruit (page 94) with soya yogurt

Wednesday

Breakfast: Green Smoothie (page 94); wholemeal toast with Salmon Pâté (page 100)

Lunch: Pasta salad made with prawns or crabmeat and Oil and Lemon Dressing (page 109); orange

Dinner: Provençal Fish (page 115) with new potatoes, cauliflower and peas; Granola (page 93) with milk and berries

Thursday

Breakfast: Grilled sardines with grilled tomatoes and mushrooms and a sliced avocado

Lunch: Home-made Hummus (page 100) with crispbread and a selection of raw vegetable sticks such as cucumber, celery and carrot; banana

Dinner: Lentil and Pea Dahl (page 126) with quinoa (page 108) and steamed broccoli; Apple Snow (page 127)

Friday

Breakfast: Fruit Smoothie (page 94); wholemeal toast with tahini and sliced tomato

Lunch: Courgette and Anchovy Pasta (page 114); grapes

Dinner: Stuffed Aubergine (page 124) with rice (page 107) and a cucumber, celery, apple and walnut salad; half a small melon

Saturday

Breakfast: Small glass fruit juice; Porridge (page 92) with sunflower and chia seeds and milk

Lunch: Crabmeat and salad with Yogurt Dressing (page 110) in wholemeal pitta bread; fresh figs or plums

Dinner: Moroccan Baked Fish with Sweet Potato Wedges (pages 115 and 105) and steamed broccoli; Pear and Carob Muffin (page 134)

Sunday

Breakfast: Bowl of wholemeal cereal with milk and raisins; wholemeal toast with Guacamole (page 101)

Lunch: Sweet Potato and Coriander Soup with Corn Bread (pages 96 and 133); fresh olives

Dinner: Baked Salmon with Roasted Summer Vegetables (pages 113 and 106) and new potatoes; Baked Banana with Cashew Nut Cream (pages 127 and 129)

Snacks

- Fruit and nut mix made of raisins, sunflower seeds, pumpkin seeds, cashew nuts and almonds.
- Raw vegetables, such as carrot sticks, celery sticks, cucumber slices, cherry tomatoes, cauliflower florets, olives. Can be eaten alone or with a dip, such as Hummus or Sardine Pâté (pages 100 and 101).
- Rice cakes or crispbread with tahini or nut butter.
- Fresh fruit, dried fruit, smoothies.

Useful addresses

Organizations and charities that offer help with diet

Allergy UK
Planwell House
LEFA Business Park
Edgington Way
Sidcup
Kent DA14 5BH
Tel.: 01322 619898 (free helpline)
Website: www.allergyuk.org

Coeliac UK
3rd Floor
Apollo Centre
Desborough Road
High Wycombe
Buckinghamshire HP11 2QW
Tel.: 01494 437278 or 0333 332
2033 (free helpline)
Website: www.coeliac.org.uk

Publishes a food and drink
directory that lists foods known to
be free of gluten, plus a magazine,
Crossed Grain, which contains
recipes and health information on
gluten-free living.

Dietary alert cards
DietaryCard
3 Inchcross Drive
Bathgate
West Lothian EH48 2HD
Tel.: 01506 635358
Website: www.dietarycard.co.uk

Produces tailor-made dietary
alert cards for people with special
dietary needs, in English or other
languages.

DIRECT-MS
5119 Brockington Road NW
Calgary, AB T2L 1R7
Canada
Website: www.direct-ms.org

The charity was founded by Dr
Ashton Embry, the originator
of the Best Bet diet. The site
includes articles on the science
behind the BBD, a link to the
BBD Diet Group's website and a
downloadable BBD recipe book.

MS Society
National Centre (MSNC)
372 Edgware Road
London NW2 6ND
Tel.: England and Wales: 020 8438
0700; Scotland: 0130 335 4050;
Northern Ireland: 02890 802802
Website: www.mssociety.org.uk

MS-UK
Unsworth House
Hythe Quay
Colchester
Essex CO2 8JF
Tel.: 01206 226500 or
0800 783 0518 (free helpline)
Website: www.ms-uk.org

As well as providing useful
information for people with
MS, this charity also publishes a
lively bi-monthly magazine, *New
Pathways*, which includes articles
on every aspect of self-help,
including diets of all kinds and
complementary therapies.

Overcoming Multiple Sclerosis
Website: www.overcomingms.org

Promotes diet and lifestyle management to improve the health and lives of people with MS. Professor George Jelinek, diagnosed with MS himself in 1999, developed his Overcoming MS Recovery programme. The website includes current research, podcasts, a community forum and details of his recovery programme.

Soil Association (England)
South Plaza
Marlborough Street
Bristol BS1 3NX
Tel.: 0117 314 5000
Website: www.soilassociation.org

Soil Association (Scotland)
3rd Floor
Osborne House
Osborne Terrace
Edinburgh EH12 5HG
Tel.: 0131 666 2474
Website: www.soilassociation.org/scotland

Both promote sustainable organic farming. Can provide details of local organic box schemes and farmers' markets.

Vegetarian Society of the United Kingdom
Parkdale
Dunham Road
Altrincham
Cheshire WA14 4QG
Tel.: 0161 925 2000
Website: www.vegsoc.org

The website has advice on vegetarian nutrition, plus a recipe section.

Organizations that promote nutritional therapy

Action on Sugar
Wolfson Institute of Preventive Medicine
Charterhouse Square
London EC1M 6BQ
Tel.: 020 7882 6219
Website: www.actiononsugar.org

British Association for Applied Nutrition and Nutritional Therapy
27 Old Gloucester Street
London WC1N 3XX
Tel.: 0870 606 1284
Website: www.bant.org.uk

This organization can help you locate a registered nutritional therapist in your area.

British Society for Ecological Medicine
3 Anson
Lower Strand
London NW9 5LT
Tel.: 07864 637723
Website: www.bsem.org.uk

The website includes a list of doctors who work in the fields of allergic, environmental and nutritional medicine.

Cambridge Nutritional Sciences
Eden Research Park
Henry Crabb Road
Littleport
Cambridgeshire CB6 1SE
Tel.: 01353 863279
Website: www.camnutri.com

This company offers the ELISA blood test for food intolerances.

NHS Smokefree
Tel.: 0300 123 1044 (free Smokefree National Helpline for England); 0800 848484 (Scotland); 0800 085 2219 (Wales); for Northern Ireland, visit website given below
Website: www.nhs.uk/smokefree; www.want2stop.info (Northern Ireland)

Companies selling useful products

Goodness Direct
South March
Daventry
Northamptonshire NN11 4PH
Tel.: 01327 701579
Website: www.goodnessdirect.co.uk

A huge range of mail-order foods for special diets available, including gluten-free, dairy-free and organic products, as well as herbal remedies and vitamin supplements.

Healthspan
PO Box 64
St Peter Port
Guernsey GY1 3BT
Tel.: 0800 7312377
Website: www.healthspan.co.uk

Supplies large range of good-quality inorganic supplements. Based in the Channel Islands, the tablets come in flat packs that pop easily through a letterbox.

Healthy Supplies
Unit 1
South Coast House
35 Chartwell Road
Lancing Business Park
Lancing
West Sussex BN15 8TU
Tel.: 0800 689 1982
Website: www.healthysupplies.co.uk

Online suppliers of foods for special diets, plus many organic and natural products.

Hydrant drinking system
Hydrate for Health Limited
1 Westfield Place
Clifton
Bristol HS8 4AY
Tel.: 0800 292 2382
Website: www.hydrateforhealth.co.uk

Hands-free drinking bottles to help avoid dehydration.

Ilumi
Thornes Business Park
Pontefract Lane
Leeds LS9 0DN
Tel.: 0800 505 3232
Website: www.ilumiworld.com

Suppliers of ready meals that are dairy-, gluten-, nut- and yeast-free and made from 100 per cent natural ingredients, all produced in the UK. A special cooking method is used, steaming the food in pouches that are then sealed and can be stored in a larder or fridge. The meals, which are reasonably priced and taste delicious, are available from Tesco and Morrisons.

Lakeland
Alexandra Buildings
Windermere
Cumbria LA23 1BQ
Tel.: 015394 88100
Website: www.lakeland.co.uk

Source of useful items for the kitchen via mail order or the company's shops across the UK.

Nature's Best
Century Place
Tunbridge Wells
Kent TN2 3BE
Tel.: 01892 552175 (nutritional advice)
Website: www.naturesbest.co.uk

Supplies organic supplements, including 1,000 iu vitamin D_3 capsules. The oil in the capsules aids absorption of their contents. All the supplements are made in the UK.

Orgran
Community Foods Limited
Brent Terrace
London NW2 1LT
Tel.: 020 8208 2966
Website: www.orgranglutenfree. co.uk

Excellent range of foods for special diets. All products are gluten-free, wheat-free, dairy-free, egg-free, yeast-free and free from artificial colours, flavours and preservatives. Bread mixes are easy to use successfully in either an oven or a breadmaker. Products are available in health food stores and online from Ocado and Goodness Direct (see page 147).

References and further reading

Brewer, Dr Sarah (2010) *The Essential Guide to Vitamins, Minerals and Herbal Supplements*. London: Robinson.

Brostoff, Professor Jonathan and Gamlin, Linda (2008) *The Complete Guide to Food Allergy and Intolerance*. London: Quality Health Books.

Davies, Dr Stephen and Stewart, Dr Alan (1987) *Nutritional Medicine*. London: Pan (although written 30 years ago, this is still the most comprehensive and reliable book on nutritional medicine I have come across).

Erasmus, Udo (1998) *Fats that Heal, Fats that Kill*. Canada: Alive Books (a thorough exploration of the role of fats in health by an internationally acclaimed expert on the subject).

Graham, Judy (2010) *Managing MS Naturally*. Vermont: Healing Arts Press.

Jelinek, Professor George (2010) *Overcoming Multiple Sclerosis: An evidence-based guide to recovery*. Lancaster: Impala Books.

Jelinek, Professor George and Law, Karen (2013) *Recovering from Multiple Sclerosis*. London: Allen & Unwin.

Swank, Roy L. and Dugan, Barbara (1987) *The MS Diet Book*. New York: Doubleday.

Wahls, Terry (2015) *The Wahls Protocol*, London: Penguin.

Recipe books and websites

Healthy eating

Over the past ten years, there has been a marked increase in cookery books promoting healthy eating and almost all the celebrity chefs have now published at least one book that falls into this category. I have found the following three useful.

Fearnley-Whittingstall, Hugh (2014) *River Cottage Light and Easy*. London: Bloomsbury.

Simple, healthy recipes, many of which use alternatives to wheat and dairy products. There is a good selection of fish and seafood dishes.

Oliver, Jamie (2015) *Everyday Superfood*. London: Michael Joseph.

Suggestions for healthy, nourishing food that is simple to make and delicious to eat.

Pinnock, Dale (2014) *Healthy Every Day: The medicinal chef*. London: Quadrille.

A food pharmacy section explains the nutrients in our food, and recipes that benefit the nervous and immune systems are clearly labelled.

Low-fat diet

BBC *Good Food* Magazine (2015) *Good Food, Eat Well: Low-fat feasts*. London: BBC Books.

<www.healthy-cooking.co.uk> This website includes low-fat Italian recipes devised by a health-conscious Italian cook. Many are also dairy- and yeast-free.

Vegan or plant-based diet

Woodward, Ella (2015) *Deliciously Ella*. London: Hodder & Stoughton.

Simple and delicious recipes for a plant-based diet by one of today's most popular food writers.

Food intolerances

There is a huge selection of books available for those coping with food intolerance, each designed to avoid different foods. Here are just two that you might find useful.

Kendrick, Pippa (2012) *The Intolerant Gourmet*. London: HarperCollins.

Recipes free of wheat, dairy, eggs and soya.

Heggie, Fiona, and Lux, Ellie (2015) *The Allergy-free Family Cookbook*. London: Orion.

Recipes free of dairy, eggs, peanuts, soya, gluten, sesame and shellfish.

The Wahls diet

Wahls, Terry (2015) *The Wahls Protocol*. London: Penguin.

Contains both recipes and menu plans.

<www.simplegreensmoothies.com> for green smoothies.

Index